How to Handle More Than You Can Handle

Caring for Yourself While Raising a Disabled Child

Amanda Griffith-Atkins, MS, LMFT

WORKMAN PUBLISHING
NEW YORK

Workman
Workman Publishing
Hachette Book Group, Inc.
1290 Avenue of the Americas
New York, NY 10104
workman.com

Workman is an imprint of Workman Publishing, a division of Hachette Book Group, Inc. The Workman name and logo are registered trademarks of Hachette Book Group, Inc.

Design by Becky Terhune

Workman books may be purchased in bulk for business, educational, or promotional use. For information, please contact your local bookseller or the Hachette Book Group Special Markets Department at special.markets@hbgusa.com.

Library of Congress Cataloging-in-Publication Data is available
ISBN 978-1-5235-2761-8

First Edition June 2025

Printed in the United States on responsibly sourced paper.

10 9 8 7 6 5 4 3 2 1

The stories and quotes in this book come from real people, or a composite of real experiences from the author's work. Some names and identifying details have been changed to protect their privacy.

For Will. It's far from perfect, but it's ours. I love you.

Contents

An Invitation to Feel

The bus pulled up in front of our Chicago two-flat, just as it did every other day. My six-year-old son slowly made his way down the bus stairs, and I met him with open arms. As we walked toward the house, he handed me his lunchbox. Inside, I found a neatly folded note from his teacher.

> *Ms. Griffith-Atkins,*
> *Would it be possible to send more food with Asher? His lunch doesn't seem to be enough. He's trying to steal other classmates' snacks after lunch and still seems hungry. He tried to take a cookie out of the trash can today.*

Rage. I crumpled up the paper. My heart pounded and I wanted to scream.

My son was born with Prader-Willi syndrome (PWS), a genetic multisystem disorder that occurs in one out of every 20,000 births. Children with PWS experience significant cognitive and physical delays, sleep disorders, infertility, and behavioral issues. But the most distinctive characteristic of this syndrome is extreme, insatiable hunger.

People with PWS can, and will, eat to the point of stomach rupture if left unattended around food. That means refrigerators and cabinets must be locked, pet food must be hidden, and toothpaste, medicine, and anything even remotely edible are potential risks.

I wanted to fire off an angry email, but, as I had so many times before, I channeled my patience. The teacher wasn't a bad person—it's our primal urge to meet a child's basic needs, especially hunger. My son was one child in a sea of thousands of hungry kids in the Chicago Public School system, although he was likely his teacher's first student to have a genetic syndrome that caused insatiable hunger. Even though Asher's needs were clearly written in his IEP (individualized education plan), and even though I'd given her a detailed document outlining his syndrome on the first day of school, the teacher obviously didn't understand the extent of his disability. So I found myself writing yet another email explaining why, no, I couldn't send more food with my son. I did my best to check my emotions for long enough to calmly educate the teacher, hoping that maybe this time she would get it. And all might be fine for a while, until a new teacher would inevitably come along and I'd have to write the email again.

When the wave of anger had passed, I did what I always tell my clients to do and unpacked the feelings. Was it *really* rage I was feeling? Or was it a deep sense of loneliness and misunderstanding? How much of my feeling was a longing for a parenting experience that included predictable milestones and "normal" challenges? My life had become rare, and it was pretty lonely being rare.

. . .

I was twenty-six years old when I gave birth to Asher. He spent a month in the NICU (neonatal intensive care unit) and then, at seven weeks old, received his diagnosis of Prader-Willi syndrome. I quickly realized that there wasn't much tolerance for conversations about the grief that comes with parenting a disabled child with high support needs. Early on, I could feel the pity and discomfort anytime I spoke of my struggles. Most people responded with encouragement, but underneath their clichéd responses was the unspoken thought: "I'm glad that didn't happen to me." I often couldn't relate to the experiences of parents of nondisabled kids, and I found myself searching for people who really understood my life as Asher's mom. I felt solidarity with disabled people but knew that they weren't the appropriate group for me to process my experience of parenting. It wasn't until I began connecting with other parents of disabled children, online and in person, that I really began to feel less alone—like I wasn't the only person in the world whose kid had a feeding tube or more specialists than friends. Eventually, rare didn't feel quite so rare after all.

There would be certain moments of clarity between us parents:

Wait, you feel that way too?

I thought I was the only one who's experienced this!

It's okay that you feel angry. I'm angry too.

I came to see how our need to appease society's expectations of what it means to be a "disability warrior"—always brave, always a fighter, always grateful—was encouraging us to bury our hard feelings even deeper.

As a trained marriage and family therapist, I knew I could use my education to help parents become healthier versions of themselves. So, after having two kids and being a stay-at-home mom for three years, I decided it was time to go back to work at the career that had meant so much to me prior to being the mom to a disabled child. I joined a practice and eventually found the confidence to launch my own practice when Asher was seven years old. From there, my business blossomed and grew into a vibrant group practice, collectively offering thousands of sessions each year to Chicagoans and beyond.

I also extended my therapy practice to parents raising disabled kids with high support needs. If you're anything like the parents I meet with every week, you have safely tucked away hard feelings about parenting a disabled child because the last thing you want is for someone to view you as a victim of your child's diagnosis (which you're not!). You may prefer to push those feelings of anger, jealousy, anxiety, and grief out of sight. That's a survival skill you've developed over time, and it's likely served you well. There's no time for a mental breakdown, right? But burying your feelings—the complicated ones, the ones that keep you up at night, the ones you're afraid to give voice to—can really take a toll. These feelings are scary to face, but by pushing them down, we're doing more harm than good.

Shortly after launching my group practice, it dawned on me that I wasn't the only parent who had complex feelings about parenting, so I turned to social media to find community. As it turns out, there were thousands of us who held shame about our emotions *and* would fight like hell to get our kid what they needed. I quickly realized that for many parents of disabled children, love and grief coexist in a muddled

These Are Our Feelings, Not Theirs

Shame, grief, fear—these feelings are valid, but when not fully understood they can move into murky territory, fraught with ableism. We can feel shame about our feelings, but not about our child. We can grieve our child's diagnosis, but not at the expense of celebrating difference. My son knows he's loved and celebrated, and I can, in good conscience, acknowledge that I grieve that the world is not always safe for him. We can feel overwhelmed by the work of caring for our child while never conveying to our child that they are a burden. I grieve the fact that my son is not able to verbally express all his emotions. I grieve that he will likely never get married or have children. Does he grieve these things? I'm not sure. And that's an important distinction to make. A diagnosis or disability is not something that inherently requires grief. There are many disabled people who do not grieve their diagnosis. My emotions are mine, and I never want to project them onto Asher. This is why we need to do the hard work of sorting our feelings—so our kids never question their worth or ability to be loved. Walking those lines takes a clear head, not one that's weighed down by unexamined feelings.

mess of emotion. I started to see my job as helping parents untangle that mess and accept and make sense of their emotions. I committed to creating space for the "dark side" of our parenting experiences where we could be vocal about our feelings—our grief, our anger, our frustrations, and more.

In therapy, the most affirming and transformative moments occur when a client sitting across from me shares the thoughts they view as shameful—usually something like "I wish my child wasn't disabled" or "I feel like I've lost myself." As a parent who's had similar thoughts, I'm able to help them shift their shame into self-compassion, give them tools to handle their emotions and relationships, and remind them that good parents don't always feel good about parenting. When we face our emotions with compassion and curiosity instead of shame and judgment, we're able to become less reactive, more self-aware versions of ourselves.

This book is an invitation to feel without apology. Studies show that if you label your emotion, your brain responds by releasing neurotransmitters that soothe your entire system. Psychiatrist Daniel Siegel coined the phrase "name it to tame it"—in other words, simply naming an emotion (saying to yourself, "I feel grief/sadness in this moment") allows your brain to take care of you. But as simple as it may be for your brain, saying the words out loud can be surprisingly hard to do.

So I'll start.

My son Asher was born with a disability that impacts his cognition, physical abilities, and communication and dramatically affects how we function as a family. He has high support needs and will require a full-time caretaker for his whole life. Since he was born, I have felt grief—both for a version of the future I had always imagined for myself and for the one I imagined for my child. I've felt helplessness—both while waiting for a proper diagnosis and then in trying to find competent and compassionate care after the diagnosis. I've felt incredible loneliness, unable to relate to the parenting experiences of my closest friends and family. I've felt rage—often!—at the world that is not built for my son and others like him. I've felt fear—mostly about the future and who will be there to take care of Asher after I'm no longer able to.

I've also felt hope, happiness, and determination. I've accepted these opposing emotions. But it started with the hard work of letting go of shame about my struggles and embracing how having a disabled child has changed me.

Because the question is not *if* parenting a disabled child will change you, it's *how*. Will you be someone who throws themselves so fully into the role of caretaker that you lose sight of who you are at your core? Will you allow anger and envy to make you a jaded version of yourself? Will you be riddled by anxiety, unable to find any semblance of hope and joy? Or will you face your emotions with tenderness to become kinder, more authentic, and accepting? My hope is for the latter—and that this book can be your companion as you work toward acceptance and self-compassion.

Some Important Notes on Language

Language is always evolving—and often limited. When I was a kid, *special needs* was the accepted term to describe disability, but using that euphemism sent the message that *disabled* was a bad word, which further suggested that disabilities are something to hide or be ashamed of. Thanks to the efforts of disability advocates, we are beginning to view disability in a more neutral way, not as a negative or a positive, but just as something that is part of the diverse landscape of being human. Because of that, I will be following the lead of disabled activists and adults and using the word *disabled*.

Moreover, I will be using the term *disabled child*, rather than *child with a disability*. For a long time, person-first language was preferred, but the shift to identity-first language, prioritizing the identity of being disabled, can be empowering. A disability is an integral part of what makes someone who they are.

Disability is a very broad term that encompasses many different meanings. According to the Americans with Disabilities Act, a disability is a physical or mental impairment that substantially limits one or more major life activities. Having a child with a disability means that their condition (mental or physical), impacts their life (and probably yours) in big ways. As you read this book, there may be examples that don't resemble your child's disability. Your child may have different medical or mobility abilities. I encourage you to take what you need from this book and consider your situation as you read about the experiences and emotions of other parents.

Now, what about terminology describing the parents of disabled children? The term *special-needs parenting* can feel like we're tiptoeing around the word *disabled*, although many parents still feel comfortable using it. *Disability parent* is another common term, but it is also complicated. *Disability parent* is an example of identity-first language, and parents can't take on the disabled identity if they themselves are not disabled. A disabled adult once said to me, "My husband doesn't call himself a disability husband because he's married to someone with a disability." There is no perfect term for us, the parents of disabled children, so I'll do the best within the limitations of the English language. In this book, you will mostly see "parent of a disabled child" or simply "parent" or "caregiver."

Last, in this book you'll see references to different levels of support needs, which can give context around a child's disability and the amount of caretaking required to keep the child safe. A person with low support needs requires mild support to get through their day. A person with high support needs *may* require assistance using the bathroom, communicating, getting dressed, and eating and likely cannot live independently. People with high support needs generally require full-time care and support.

I wrote this book primarily for fellow parents of children with high support needs, with the understanding that there would be plenty that resonates with parents of children with low or moderate support needs. In this book, you'll hear from parents whose kids have diagnoses that run the gamut, but most of their children require a high level of parental involvement to help them function throughout the day. (Most names have been changed to protect their children's privacy.) There is no one-size-fits-all approach to raising disabled kids, and that includes the advice given in parenting books. I hope you will take what feels relevant to your family and leave the rest.

A Scary and Sacred Job

My disabled son has changed my life for the better. Knowing him and seeing life through his eyes has reminded me of what's important and given me a perspective I wish the whole world shared. I've learned to value every single day with him and not take health for granted. I've grown to see every chromosome as something to be thankful for and now believe that it's a true miracle that so many of us are walking around with forty-six of them, each fully intact. As we make space for our struggles, we open ourselves up to see the beauty and diversity in

Listening to Disabled Voices

Ashley Harris Whaley is a disabled activist and speaker. When asked what her number one piece of advice would be for the parents of disabled children, Ashley said, "Become educated on disability."

Ashley encourages parents to consume a broad representation of information produced by disabled people. This will not only educate us but keep us attuned with disabled activists, ensuring that we're challenging our own internalized ableism. Many valuable resources are available, such as books, podcasts, and social media accounts.

Ashley emphasizes a crucial detail: As nondisabled parents of disabled children, we must actively seek wisdom from disabled individuals. This approach will not only enlighten us but also empower us to better support our children.

Ashley said, "Having a disabled kid doesn't automatically make you an ally. The representation and education piece is a huge part of allyship."

disability. Part of our work is seeing that beauty and struggle can coexist in a stunning shade of gray. It's not good or bad—it simply is.

In her book *Disability Visibility*, activist Alice Wong writes, "Disability is mutable and ever evolving. Disability is both apparent and nonapparent. Disability is pain, struggle, brilliance, abundance, and joy. Disability is sociopolitical, cultural, and biological. Being visible and claiming a disabled identity brings risks as much as it brings pride."

I can almost taste Wong's words. I can feel the depth and vastness of what it means to live life alongside my disabled child. As we parent and care for our disabled children, we experience the full essence of disability. We experience such an intimate connection to disability yet aren't disabled. We are caretakers and parents of disabled children, and that is a scary and sacred job. Depending on our child's disability, we may be entrusted to make decisions on their behalf. We cannot do that in good and clear conscience unless we face our emotions about this role.

My fellow caretakers, we have a big task ahead of us. My hope is that this book will unravel all the unspoken feelings inside you and give you a place to make sense of all the emotions you feel like you're not allowed to feel. Up until now, there hasn't been much of a forum for us to work through our shit together. The goal of digging into the hard stuff isn't to say woe is me or complain about our lives; it's to collectively face our experiences with the goal of coming out as better humans and parents. You deserve to function out of survival mode. Do you need to read that again? *You deserve to function out of survival mode.* My hope is that you find the safety, self-compassion, and grace you need to return to (or, in some cases, to rediscover) yourself as a person, not just as a parent hanging on for dear life.

If I tell you to do it for your child, I know you will. But I won't say that because if you're anything like me, you probably do everything for your child. Let this commitment to emotional exploration be a radical act of self-care, because when it's all said and done, you're worth it.

1

Parent Meets Kid

CHAPTER 1

First Feelings

I don't remember the theme of my baby shower, but I do remember it being lovely and thoughtfully planned. Every little detail was perfect. I wore a long brown empire-waist dress that highlighted my pregnant belly, and I joyfully posed for pictures with each of the guests who attended. I was one of the first of my friends to get pregnant, and I teased them that their day was coming. They smiled at the thought. I opened each gift and held up each perfect outfit and brightly colored children's book. *Oh, a blanket! And thank you! A nursing pillow!*

"Will you be trying for a natural birth?" one friend asked.

The answer was yes. I had done my research and concluded that a "natural" birth was best. I wanted as little intervention as possible and skin-to-skin contact right away. I selected a smaller community hospital closer to our home instead of the mammoth, fancy downtown hospital where epidurals were given like candy and cesareans were conducted on assembly lines. (And yes, I secretly judged the women who chose to deliver there.)

When I was just over thirty-six weeks pregnant, my doctor made the decision to induce me. The baby was measuring small and there were concerns about the placenta, but I wasn't too worried. It was April in Chicago, and the forecast was calling for unseasonably warm temperatures and bright blue skies. I'll never forget my doctor saying to me, "You'll be holding your baby on the porch by the weekend!"

It sounded perfect, holding my baby on the back porch of our small Chicago condo. I knew the early delivery wasn't ideal, but I was ready for this pregnancy to be over and to hold my baby in my arms. My biggest fear was that I might have to get a C-section, but I was committed to doing everything in my power to avoid it.

As it turns out, the C-section would be the least of my concerns. Instead, I was begging God or the Universe or anyone who would listen to just let my baby live. It was my first experience with the now familiar, always painful reality for many parents of disabled kids: the moving of the goalposts. Instead of dreaming about what our children will become when they grow up, we dream that they get to grow up. Instead of hoping for high test scores, we hope for normal bloodwork, clear MRIs, or normal genetic testing. My baby needed a small part of his fifteenth chromosome and a feeding tube, not a $2,000 stroller.

Somehow, the Earth keeps turning even when our world comes to a crashing halt. While Asher was in the NICU, my parents were staying with me and my husband to offer support. One evening we decided to try to take a mental break from the roller coaster of the NICU and go out for dinner.

"Where should we eat?" someone said.

Is my baby going to die? I thought.

"Does Mexican sound good?" someone else added.

What will our future look like? I wondered.

At the restaurant, I wondered what people saw when they looked at us. Could they tell I had just given birth? I still looked pregnant, the way mothers naturally do after they give birth. My milk had come in and my breasts were engorged. As the waitress took our order, I wanted to scream at her: *Do you know what has happened to me?* How could she act so normal when my world felt completely shattered?

Giving birth to a disabled child or finding out that your child has become disabled can be, at the very least, emotionally shattering and, at most, deeply traumatic. In this chapter, I'm going to walk you through some of the most common hard feelings that new parents of disabled children experience. For me, those feelings included jealousy, anger, helplessness, and a sense that I wasn't a real parent. And yes, some very real trauma. Whether your child was born disabled or became disabled later, my guess is you have your own story filled with complex emotions and experience. Our stories may be different, but we likely share similar emotions.

Feeling Helpless

If your child is born prematurely or medically fragile (as many disabled children are), you're likely familiar with the neonatal intensive care unit. You very quickly become acclimated to the smells, sounds, and sights of your baby's temporary home. Every day a new specialist is poking and prodding at your baby, and for many new parents, each moment is filled with dread, anxiety, helplessness, and trauma.

"I was her mother, and I couldn't help her," said Angela as she reflected on her daughter Helena's 101 days in the NICU. "Those first weeks consisted of a revolving door of different specialists coming in to deliver bad news on top of bad news. So often, I had the urge to run out the double doors. I didn't want to be there, and at the same time, it hurt like hell to leave my daughter at the end of every day. I was afraid that something terrible might happen and I wouldn't be there."

Of course, anyone, at any age, can become disabled. There's a unique type of grief that comes from witnessing your child lose certain abilities and needing to relearn how to exist in the world with a body or mind that doesn't function like it used to.

Allie Wade was a typically developing, active five-year-old girl when she fell off a couch and landed on her head, which resulted in a stroke, likely from an undiagnosed brain malformation. The stroke left Allie paralyzed from the neck down, a condition that will likely last for the rest of her life. After six months spent in the hospital, she eventually returned home reliant on a trach tube, ventilator, pacemaker, G-tube, and wheelchair. All of this happened at the height of the COVID-19 pandemic, which was an added layer of risk and complication.

"Going through something like this feels like bricks sitting on your chest. It's a horrible, horrible feeling," said Allie's mom, Deonna, as she reflected on the experience of seeing Allie fight for her life. "It's all made me care about very little, and for the most part, I love that perspective, but I also have PTSD, depression, and anxiety from the entire experience."

And who could blame her? Watching your child go from walking, talking, and laughing to being reliant on caregivers for everything is a devastating process. Overnight, Deonna's sense of safety and predictability was shattered.

I have vivid memories from Asher's NICU stay, each day bringing a new hypothesis of what was going on with him. He was having a hard time breathing—did he need plastic surgery to correct his recessed chin? Was he simply premature and just needed some time to catch up? Or was it a genetic condition called Prader-Willi syndrome? Asher had every single presenting symptom for Prader-Willi syndrome (PWS)— we just needed genetic testing to confirm. We held on to hope that Asher's condition was something that could be corrected with time or even a surgery. Sometimes hope is the only thing you have while your child is hospitalized.

After a few days, I was discharged from the hospital, while Asher stayed in the NICU. My husband and I began to settle into life as new parents. The only thing missing was the baby. Each night, my husband would call the hospital to check on Asher. It was like getting a daily report from daycare, only instead of hearing about diaper changes and nap schedules we were talking about oxygen levels, tolerating eating, and breathing patterns. This became our new normal. I'd wake up multiple times in the middle of the night to pump because it felt like the only thing I could do to care for my baby while he was in the NICU.

Every morning at 3 a.m., I would sit in the living room and pump, watching out my window as the newspaper delivery truck pulled up to the L train station across the street. The delivery person, illuminated by the streetlights, would unload a stack of newspapers and put them in the dispenser in preparation for the morning commuters, while I sat there listening to the "wickie, wickie, wickie" whir of the pump on repeat. It wasn't how I had envisioned motherhood, but it was my reality.

Sheena gave birth to a micropreemie who weighed 1.35 pounds at birth. Her daughter was later diagnosed with spastic diplegic cerebral palsy.

"It was the hardest, most gut-wrenching experience of my life. Nothing could have prepared me for it," Sheena reflected. "I felt so empty. I remember the first night after I gave birth. She had been intubated and whisked away. I was terrified."

Research has consistently shown that NICU parents are at a high risk for postpartum mood disorders. A 2010 study discovered that parents of babies who spent time in the NICU are 40 percent more likely to develop postpartum depression than parents of healthy babies. The study found various reasons for this increased risk: the emotional toll of having a medically fragile baby, the financial stress of a long NICU stay, the noises, the stressful environment, even the lack of natural sunlight. Many parents report feeling a deep sense of helplessness while their child is in the NICU, in part because there's just not much they can do to care for their baby. Most parents instinctively respond to their baby's cues: baby cries, baby is fed. But in the NICU, a baby's needs are far beyond what a parent can meet, and the stakes are incredibly high.

Feeling Unneeded and Detached

Watching at team of medical experts take care of your newborn baby can feel crushing. This can lead to a parent feeling unneeded and maybe even detached.

In the NICU, it's easy to feel robbed of the special moments that build our confidence as new parents. Instead of our clumsy and sometimes laughable first diaper change, a nurse swiftly swaps diapers, mindful of keeping all the necessary wires attached. For more seasoned parents, it's frustrating to feel sidelined by doctors, almost as if you, the parent, are not needed.

"I felt like a part-time mom, or a mom on paper and in spirit but not in real life," said Sheena. "I didn't know what my daughter liked or what her normal schedule was. I focused a lot on pumping because that was the only 'mom thing' I could consistently do. Pumping was the only steady connection I had to being a mom. Everything else—holding her, changing her diaper, or bathing her—was dependent on her health that day or a schedule."

When you have a child who depends on therapists, specialists, nurses, and machines for survival, it's easy to feel like you're not needed. Whether your child is in the NICU or admitted to the hospital at any age, it's important to remember that you are irreplaceable as their parent. Your child needs nurturing, safety, and consistency, all of which you are fully capable of providing. Lean into the moments of parenting that help you feel most connected to your child. This might look like reading a book bedside in the hospital, providing a bedtime routine in between vitals and medications, or making a point to take your child out of their hospital room if possible (for a walk in the hallway or just anywhere to get a change of scenery). Above all, your child deserves the normalcy that you can provide as their parent. When Asher was in the NICU, I brought children's books to read to him because it felt like something "real moms" got to do. Don't underestimate the power of finding simple ways to connect with your child while they are in the hospital.

The stress of having a child in the hospital is immense. It's easy to feel burned out as the weight of the world accumulates on your shoulders. You might be worrying about the future (how will we ever adjust to caretaking at home?), feeling guilty for the responsibilities you're not tending to (like work or your other children), or just longing for a moment to yourself to rest and decompress. These are very real worries and feelings. You are not a one-dimensional person and you have a full, complex life. Putting your life on hold for an extended period is never easy. It is important (and completely appropriate) for you to take breaks from the hospital. Go home, shower, move your body, sleep in your own bed. Be intentional about eating something other than hospital food. You cannot show up day after day at the hospital without fueling yourself physically, emotionally, and spiritually. Reach out to your support system. Ask your best friend or a family member to rally your friends and family to provide meals, help care for your other children, or even come sit with your child while you get a break for an afternoon. Above all, give yourself permission to accept help when it's offered.

Feeling Jealous

The disconnect between other parents and me started the day Asher was born, but the first time I really felt that pang of jealously was four days after Asher's birth. I was sitting by his crib in the NICU scrolling through Facebook when I came across a picture of an old college friend holding her healthy newborn. She looked more beautiful and happier than ever, tears in her eyes as she held her precious baby. Meanwhile, my baby was hooked up to no less than ten cords, each connected to a mind-blowingly expensive piece of equipment that startled me every time it beeped. Then, a few days later, that same friend lamented online about how she wasn't getting any sleep. My child was being cared for around the clock by nurses, and here I was, fully rested and feeling nothing like a mother. Overnight, light-years had grown between my friend's experience and my own—suddenly I didn't know where I belonged. I was also really jealous.

Asher was in the NICU for nearly a month. I remember one late-night drive home from the hospital. My husband clicked the windshield wipers up to the highest setting as the rain pounded down outside. While stopped at a traffic light, I looked out the window and saw what I believed to be a very young mother walking in the rain with her baby in a stroller. Rain fell hard on her and on her tiny baby, and I began to tell myself the story of how her baby was perfectly healthy and she didn't even know how lucky she was. Grief washed over me, quickly turning to indignation. Why did *she* get to have a healthy baby? I would never take my baby out in the rain. Life felt so unfair.

I felt so jealous of all my friends who had an easy birthing experience and a nondisabled newborn. It felt like everyone else gave birth to a healthy baby. I was jealous that my friends were up all night with a crying baby and that they got to go to Mommy & Me classes. I was ashamed of this feeling—jealousy felt so ugly and petty. I also felt guilty because I knew my friends would be hurt if they knew how I felt. I judged myself for feeling such a toxic emotion, even though I knew there are no bad feelings and jealousy is a perfectly healthy emotion. I look back at that younger version of myself and I feel compassion.

If you have wrestled with jealousy, extend some compassion to yourself and acknowledge the pain behind the feeling. Imagine a conversation with your jealousy, where you speak directly to it. Perhaps you'd say something like, "You're here because it's painful to see everyone else have what you want." Approach your feelings of jealousy with kindness.

It's also important to consider how you relate to the people you feel jealousy toward. It's okay to take some distance from them, but be up front about it. Let your friends know that it's just too painful to be around them right now and that it's nothing they did. Or say that you'd love to hang out, but you just can't talk about your birth experience yet. Your clear communication will help your loved ones care for you and help preserve your relationship during this difficult time.

Feeling Overwhelmed

Eventually, be it two days, two weeks, six months, or somewhere in between, you will bring your child home from the hospital. It will be both terrifying and joyful. There will likely still be many unanswered questions about what the future will bring, but one thing will be certain—your new normal has begun.

"Coming home from the NICU was simultaneously the most terrifying and thrilling day of my life," said Lauren. "I could not believe my daughter was finally mine. I was so excited for her to sleep in her crib and be rocked in the chair I picked out. But also, I couldn't believe I was solely responsible for her care. What if an emergency happened? I had a hard time cutting off her hospital bracelet because I was scared we'd have to return back."

When was that moment for you? When the institution that once held you suddenly let you go out into the world on your own, did you feel like you were drowning? The life jacket that once kept you afloat is suddenly stripped away. This transition is both terrifying and empowering, and for some, the former feels much stronger.

"My daughter was born nondisabled but was left with cognitive impairment after surviving a brain tumor," Frank said. "We had been through so much and were grateful Isabell survived, but she was basically a different person from who she used to be. We began to realize that even though she survived a brain tumor, life would never go back to the way it used to be."

Coming home with a child who requires extra care has the potential to challenge every single part of your life. The transition to parenting your child may now include tasks and responsibilities that you never imagined needing to prepare for. We all enter parenthood expecting to change diapers, but changing a gastrostomy tube? Not so much. At the same time, the other demands of life don't just go away. We eventually must return to work, clean our homes, parent our other children, and reengage with our loved ones.

Especially in the beginning, managing the responsibilities of caring

Five Tips for Finding Peace Post-NICU

1. Share your child's journey. When Asher came home from the NICU with a nasogastric (NG) tube, I hesitated to take pictures. His appearance was different from that of other babies, but his NG tube was part of his unique story. Looking back, I wish I had shared his journey earlier. Embrace your child's uniqueness and share their story with your loved ones. Your community is eager to see your beautiful baby, so don't keep them hidden.

2. Practice self-compassion. It's crucial to be kind to yourself as you navigate the challenges of raising a disabled child. If you need one, place a reminder on your bathroom mirror that says, "One day at a time." Remember, it's okay to take time to adjust to your new normal. Your mental and physical well-being are important, especially when you're adjusting to your child's ongoing health concerns.

3. When you're ready, connect with other parents of disabled children (more on this later). Community will continue to be your lifeline and being around other disabled children and their parents can be incredibly healing. You are not alone in this journey, and there are others who understand and can support you.

4. Find ways to physically connect with your child. Asher's NG tube required extra attention whenever I picked him up. I noticed some people were hesitant to pick him up, so I always made a point to invite loved ones to hold him.

5. Pay attention to the moments when you feel most yourself. It's easy to lose connection with who you are when you're thrown into the world of parenting a disabled child. If you love running, try to prioritize getting out a couple of times a week for a jog. Your hobbies matter and knowing what brings you joy is essential to your sense of self. Remember, taking care of yourself is not a luxury, it's a necessity.

for a disabled child can feel so overwhelming. You must be gentle with yourself (am I sounding like a broken record yet?). You're not a robot, and it's important that you take things day by day and acknowledge your needs and limits. Some people prefer to jump back into work or life commitments because it helps them find familiarity amid the new responsibilities that might come with having a disabled child. Others prefer to have everything come to a halt while they assume the role of primary caretaker to their child. How you integrate back into the real world will impact your relationships, and it's important to acknowledge your emotions and needs, especially with your partner. Year one of parenting very quickly turns into year two and three, and before you know it patterns are set in place that impact your marriage and your other children. I say this to encourage you to be open and curious about the way you handle your reentry to the real world after you become the parent to a disabled child. You're setting the scene for how you function in the future.

Understanding Trauma

For many of you, these early days and first feelings may have been years, if not decades ago. But if you're anything like me, the smell of hospital soap can take you right back to that scary time. Watching your child go through a medical emergency or catastrophic experience at any age is enough to leave anyone traumatized. Research suggests that at least 60 percent of parents who had a baby in the NICU experience post-traumatic stress disorder (PTSD). Many parents of disabled kids also suffer from acute trauma disorder (ATD), a condition that can develop right after seeing a traumatic event, such as witnessing your child being resuscitated, having a seizure, or struggling to breathe.

In an interview with *The Guardian*, physician and trauma expert Gabor Maté said, "Trauma is not what happens to you; it is what happens inside you as a result of what happens to you." When you have a child who is in and out of the hospital or who is medically fragile,

What Is PTSD?

The term PTSD gets thrown around a lot ("That scary movie gave me PTSD!" "I have PTSD from that last workout!"), but what is post-traumatic stress disorder, for real? The *DSM-5-TR* is a handbook used by mental health professionals in the United States that classifies mental disorders. Its criteria for a PTSD diagnosis is as follows:

1. A person has been exposed to a stressor in the following ways: It happened to them, they witnessed it happen to someone else, they learned that a loved one was exposed to a trauma, or they were indirectly exposed to details of the trauma.

2. The person experiences at least one of the following intrusive symptoms: upsetting memories, nightmares, flashbacks, emotional reaction after being exposed to reminders of the traumatic event, or physical response after being exposed to reminders of the traumatic event.

3. The person avoids thinking about the trauma or anything that could provoke reminders of the trauma.

4. The person is experiencing negative thoughts or moods because of the trauma.

5. The person is experiencing negative physical sensations as a result of the trauma, such as irritability, depression, difficulty sleeping, hypervigilance, or heightened startle response.

potential trauma triggers are everywhere. It's not uncommon for a disabled child to struggle to breathe or go through a painful procedure, or for their parents to have huge emotional swings arising from the information they're given each day. These scary experiences stick with us long after we've lived them in real life.

So, what exactly happens in your brain when you're experiencing trauma? First, let's explore how memories are made and stored in the body. Imagine yourself in a beautiful flower garden. Perhaps you pass a gorgeous lilac blush in full bloom, with its sweet scent filling the air. You see the light purple blooms and even reach out to touch them, noticing that they're soft and fragile. When you go home that night, you have a vivid image in your head of what you saw that day and may even be able to conjure up a soft scent of lilacs. Over time, however, the somatic experience of the flower garden fades. You won't be able to remember the way the flowers looked and smelled in the same way you did right after you saw them. After a few days, the memory shifts from something that you can relive with your senses to a factual experience that lives in your brain. In other words, you will be able to recall that the flowers were beautiful and smelled lovely, but you won't be able to conjure up the smell the way you did a few days earlier. Your brain does this to keep you in the present moment and help you distinguish a memory from the here and now.

Traumatic experiences are not processed in the same way as pleasant or everyday experiences. Traumatic experiences (which can mean different things for different people) do not go through the process of being turned into facts. They get stuck in the here and now.

Therapist Kayleigh Summers, known as the Birth Trauma Mama on social media, has spent her career focusing on birth trauma. "A brain imaging study was done that showed what happens when trauma is activated. As it turns out, trauma is experienced by the brain as a present event rather than a memory. This means every time your trauma is activated, your nervous system goes into fight, flight, freeze, or fawn mode. You don't have control over this, it is an automatic response," she explained. "This is why so often after trauma, survivors feel like they're waiting for the other shoe to drop. It's not just worry, it's that their nervous system genuinely believes a trauma is about to happen again."

So, that feeling of dread? You're not making it up. You're probably not overreacting. Your brain thinks that a horrifying event that happened days, weeks, months, or even years ago is happening right now. And here's something else to note: Because trauma is so all-encompassing for your nervous system, it's difficult to process any

The Four Fs of Trauma Response, Explained

When you're faced with a traumatic trigger, your body automatically responds in one of four ways. The main goal of this response is to keep you safe from the perceived threat. Let's say you're swimming in the ocean and you spot a shark close by. How might you respond?

- Flight—You're out of there! You swim to safety as quickly as possible.

- Fight—There's no time to get away so you do all you can to fight the shark off.

- Freeze—Your body shuts down and you can't think or move. You play dead, hoping that the shark will be uninterested and move on to its next victim.

- Fawn—You decide to try to keep the shark happy by playing with it in the water and keeping it entertained.

It's important to add that weeks later, when you walk by the ocean again, you might start to panic because your brain brings you right back to the time when you almost got attacked by a shark. Your trauma response (fight, flight, freeze, or fawn) may kick in even though you're not actually in danger.

other emotions (such as grief!) when you're living in a traumatized state. Don't be surprised if you suddenly become aware of feelings of grief once you've begun healing from trauma.

Licensed marriage and family therapist and trauma therapist Tovah Means knows firsthand what it's like to experience a traumatic birth and have a baby in the NICU. She gave birth to her daughter Luna at thirty-four weeks of gestation. Luna spent four weeks in the NICU, and while the medical staff made the hospitalization as positive as possible, Tovah felt disconnected from much of the experience.

"You're in fight-or-flight mode, your heart is racing, your mind is spinning, you can't sleep," she recalled. "These are all normal PTSD reactions. Your body's just waiting for the determining factor, which is either my baby is going to survive or they are not."

Tovah noted that it's important for a traumatized parent to get support as soon as they get home with their baby: "If at all possible, try not to be alone. Make sure there's someone getting things ready for you at home. You need to sleep, eat, and get support around you because it's so overwhelming."

When I was with Asher in the NICU, the wife of a Major League Baseball player often sat next to me. We'd make small talk about our babies or ourselves.

"How long have you been in here?"

"Does your baby have a diagnosis?"

"How is she doing today?"

This started to feel like my own version of the park or library: just two new parents chatting about their children. This setting wasn't quite as peaceful, but I was thankful to have someone to talk with to make the hours pass.

As humans, we're wired for intergenerational support and crave mentoring from someone who has experienced what we've been through. This innate need for wisdom highlights the importance of community. If you know someone who has brought a baby home from the NICU, it might be helpful to reach out to them. Or you can look for support online, among the communities of people who have a similar experience and get what you're going through. Whatever you do, don't navigate your first few weeks home from the NICU alone.

"You're so tired that you're not able to look out for yourself. Your support system can notice if you're not handling things successfully with your baby," Tovah said.

The Power of Therapy

After twenty-two days in the NICU and an emotionally draining pregnancy, Madeline Cheney found herself in therapy to address sleep problems that she thought stemmed from grief from the loss of her father, who had died when she was young. Very quickly, the therapist gently suggested that Madeline was struggling with trauma from having a child with a life-changing disability. Madeline's son Kimball was born with a rare genetic syndrome called X-linked chondrodysplasia punctata 1 (CDPX1), which has approximately 125 known documented cases. Madeline and her therapist began EMDR (eye movement desensitization and reprocessing) therapy, which utilizes bilateral brain stimulation, initiated by the therapist moving their hand, using blinking lights, or tapping. Developed by psychologist Francine Shapiro, EMDR is thought to work in the same way as REM sleep, which has a natural ability to help the brain reprocess traumatic memories.

Madeline's therapist encouraged her to pick her most traumatic memory, the one that would rank at the highest stress point. Madeline identified the initial ultrasound, when the doctor first noticed something abnormal. The ultrasound showed that Kimball had short limbs and extra amniotic fluid. The doctor was unable to discern his nose bone and said that more testing was needed to determine what was going on.

"My trauma started out like an infected wound," Madeline said.

Trauma: A Five-Sense Experience

I recently took Asher to his biannual endocrinology appointment. I took a minute to use the bathroom there, and as I washed my hands, my heart suddenly started to pound and a strong feeling of dread came over me. The smell of the antiseptic soap common in most medical offices brought my brain right back to Asher's monthlong stay in the NICU, where I was required to scrub in, soaping every inch of my arms up to my elbows multiple times per day. Research shows that scent can conjure up memories more vividly than sight. Sixteen years later, the smell of the soap brought the trauma of those weeks right into the present.

She and her therapist cleaned and rebandaged the wound week after week with EMDR.

"The reprocessing felt so painful because I was facing all of these intense, difficult memories head-on, but using EMDR helped me to feel like I could finally properly heal," Madeline added. "Now when I think about it, it's not even all negative. I'm able to remember that time in the doctor's office and begin to see it with some distance. Now I have so much self-compassion, even excitement, because I am able to see that that ultrasound represented my son. That memory morphed from a really loaded memory that felt awful into something that became special and tender. EMDR has had a domino effect that helped me gain a new perspective on everything."

The goal of any trauma therapy centers around integrating traumatic memories. Trauma therapists tend to use a bottom-up approach to access the part of the brain that stores memories, where they're stuck and fragmented. This means that a therapist may begin by helping you to understand sensations in your body, as opposed to exploring thoughts or feelings such as sadness or anger. Look for a type of therapy that prioritizes the nervous system rather than just the cognitive parts of the brain. There are several different modalities to choose from, including:

- Eye movement desensitization and reprocessing (EMDR): This therapy uses bilateral brain stimulation triggered by horizontal hand movement, blinking lights, or tapping to help a person process traumatic memories and decrease their emotional reactivity.

- Internal family systems (IFS): This form of talk therapy is based on the concept that our mind is made up of different internal parts that interact with one another much like the members of a family do. All of these parts have a role in how we function, and if we can better understand them, we can respond to our emotions with compassion.

- Polyvagal therapy: This practice focuses on the role that our automatic nervous system (especially the vagus nerve) has in self-regulation. In this therapy, clients learn exercises, such as breathwork, to help stimulate the vagus nerve and soothe their nervous system.

- Brainspotting: This mind-body therapy uses the visual field and occipital nerve to better access parts of the brain that are involved in specific distressing memories. During brainspotting, the therapist moves a pointer object in a specific pattern in front of the client's eyes. The client responds with a reflexive signal, such as an eye twitch, yawn, or facial expression, that indicates that a brainspot has been discovered. A brainspot is an eye position that correlates with where the brain is holding an emotional memory. The therapist and client then work to process the memory and correlating emotion.

• • •

The NICU was Asher's first home, but his real home was with me and his dad. After four weeks in the hospital, my baby finally came *home*. My husband and I now had the enormous responsibility of parenting a disabled child. The trauma of the NICU was just the beginning of our story, and sixteen years later I can now say that I've fostered a bond with my son, far, far away from the incessant beeping of machines and ever-present medical staff that surrounded us early on. But that bond took time, in part because we had just begun to get to know each other away from the NICU, and also because I wasn't prepared for the added responsibilities that came with caring for a medically fragile child. But Rome wasn't built overnight, and it's possible that your bond with your child won't be either.

Once we got settled at home, I went into Asher's room, opened the closet, and reached for a blanket I had folded and tucked away weeks ago. I picked up my tiny baby and rested his head in the crook of my arm. I gave myself permission, just for a moment, to forget about the pending genetic test, the "what ifs" looming over us, and just be in this present moment.

   We made our way to the porch, and I felt my shoulders drop as I inhaled the warm spring air. Finally, at long last, I sat in the sunshine with my baby.

Reflection Exercise

Parenthood is loaded with hopes and expectations. From the moment (and even before) we see a positive pregnancy test, our heads are swirling with fantasies of raising our child. Take some time to reflect on your experience. While you're answering the questions below, notice your emotions. Notice what feelings you find yourself avoiding as well as any judgment toward yourself. Remember, there are no bad feelings. The goal of this exercise is twofold: to draw meaning from your experience of becoming the parent to your child, and to become more aware of your feelings and how you respond to them.

- Can you identify your before and after of becoming the parent to your disabled child?
  - *Was your child born with a known disability?*
  - *Did it take some time for you to realize your child was disabled?*
  - *Was there an event or illness that contributed to your child's disability?*
  - *How did your unique experience of the above three questions impact your emotions?*
- Did the process of realizing your child was disabled impact your sense of safety in the world? If yes, how?

- Did you experience trauma through childbirth or the NICU?

  - *If your child wasn't in the NICU, did you experience trauma through the events that led to your child becoming disabled?*

  - *What are common trauma triggers for you?*

  - *How do/did you respond to trauma triggers? Fight, flight, freeze, or fawn?*

- What changed in your life after you became the parent to your child?

- What emotions are you noticing as you answer these questions?

CHAPTER 2

Searching for Answers

Veronica was twenty-five weeks pregnant with her third child when I received her email.

> *Dear Amanda,*
>
> *My unborn son was just diagnosed with tuberous sclerosis complex after my doctor discovered a noncancerous tumor in his heart. This is probably the first of many tumors we will find due to his condition. I know we have a long road ahead, but I don't even know where to begin.*

One week later, Veronica sat nervously on my pink couch, fidgeting with a hair tie around her wrist. If I hadn't known better, I would have assumed that Veronica was like every other woman in their second trimester—excited, hopeful, and slightly uncomfortable. But Veronica was terrified. She had spent hours googling "tuberous sclerosis complex" and quickly became an expert on the condition, yet she could not fully envision the future.

I was very familiar with this sensation.

When Asher had been home from the NICU for about three weeks, I got a call on my cell phone. I had saved this number in my phone as "Children's Genetics—Answer," so I did just that. We had been waiting for this moment for weeks.

The genetic counselor wasted no time.

"We got your son's genetic testing back and the results correlate with a syndrome."

Time. Stood. Still.

This was the moment. My heart pounded in my chest, and I felt the wind knocked out of me.

"Your son has Prader-Willi syndrome. It's caused by a defect on chromosome 15." She began to speak slowly now. "The syndrome is a multisystem disorder that impacts cognition, hormones, behavior, and development. We recommend your husband undergo genetic testing because it's usually caused by a deletion on the paternal side. We'd like to meet with you on Monday to answer any questions you might have." The geneticist spoke softly, as if her tone and pacing could somehow make the blow a little softer.

The movie *Twilight* was playing on my TV in the background as the genetic counselor explained Asher's diagnosis. I'd seen it a million times. It's a story about a human who falls in love with a vampire and struggles to maintain a relationship with her bloodthirsty boyfriend. Essentially, *Twilight* is about one girl's desperate attempts to fit into a family that could kill her. Suddenly, I began to see my son's life the same way; danger was everywhere. I remembered a physician in the hospital explaining that people with PWS cannot control their food intake and I would need to keep refrigerators locked. How would my baby survive in a world where he wouldn't be able to trust his own instincts about the very thing that sustains him? What would birthday parties or holidays look like? Could we ever eat out at restaurants? How would our friends respond to our needs? Would our families still love Asher and prioritize having a relationship with him? Even more terrifyingly, what if my child died?

"Ma'am, are you okay?" the genetic counselor asked.

"Yes. Yes, I'm okay. Thank you, have a nice day, bye." *Wait, was that how I was supposed to respond?* I hung up the phone as my world came crumbling down.

In that sliver of time, I was the only person (aside from the geneticist) who knew about the diagnosis. Other people's lives went on without disruption. Even my husband, who was working in an office ten miles away, had no idea that Asher had a life-altering diagnosis. My loved ones were at work, or making dinner, or driving, or going for

Caring for Yourself While Looking for Answers

- Tune in to how you feel as you dive into internet research. If googling leaves you feeling discouraged and hopeless, allow yourself to slow down. It's natural to want to absorb every bit of information about your child's diagnosis, but it's crucial to pace yourself to avoid feeling overwhelmed.

- Embrace moments of joy. You will likely be faced with a lot of complex emotions post-diagnosis. It's easy to withdraw and turn inward. However, it's important to intentionally seek joy to remind yourself that life isn't hopeless and there's still plenty of good in the world. Take a walk, have sex, get coffee with a friend, read a book, watch your favorite movie—it's okay to feel happiness.

- Your child's identity remains unchanged despite the diagnosis. Yes, your expectations of the future may shift, but the present is still the same. They're still your precious child, lovable and valuable. Don't let your fears of the future impact your ability to connect with your child today.

walks. I wondered how I might possibly handle the enormous responsibility of telling people what I had just been told. I felt like the doctor had thrown a bomb at me and I had to pass it on to someone else before it destroyed me.

As my mind raced, I stared down at my beautiful eight-pound baby. He was snuggled cozily into the couch, fingers twitching as he slept, without a care in the world. As a breeze from the open window behind us stirred his wispy blonde hair, I nuzzled my nose into his cheek and breathed in his smell. For the first time, two truths began to form in my mind, and though they seemed to oppose themselves at first, I forced them to sit comfortably together; in the months that followed, I'd become adept at this particular skill. The first truth: My newborn baby was precious and perfect. The second? My newborn baby had a rare genetic syndrome that would forever change the course of our lives.

At twenty-six, I was faced with the reality that I would be a caretaker until the end of my life, or his, whichever came first. The parenting journey I had envisioned was now a path to be reimagined, one where I would learn to embrace and eventually celebrate my child's unique needs and personality. But before the celebration, I would need time for recovery, self-compassion, and for the emotional dust to settle.

Feeling Guilty, Learning to Forgive

Natalie, mom to Cara, found herself going from specialist to specialist, desperately seeking answers. Natalie, like most parents, initially brought her concerns to her pediatrician, who incorrectly diagnosed her daughter with Rett syndrome. From there, genetic testing was done and a rare microduplication was confirmed. Natalie feared the microduplication was just a piece of the puzzle, though, and she continued to seek opinions from specialists.

Prompted by Cara's unusual movements when she woke up from naps, Natalie made an appointment to see a neurologist. Her hopes of finding answers were quickly crushed when the neurologist dismissed her concerns. "I felt like an idiot the way she brushed me off and rushed us out of the door. Our appointment was ten minutes long," Natalie remembered.

Back to the drawing board, Natalie was finally able to schedule an appointment with a geneticist. "Within two minutes of our appointment, the doctor noticed that Cara was having tremors, something the therapists, other neurologists, and I had not noticed."

This, along with the other information Natalie shared, prompted the geneticist to refer Cara to yet another neurologist. Two weeks later Cara had an EEG, was admitted to the hospital, and got a confirmed diagnosis of Lennox-Gastaut syndrome, a severe form of epilepsy. The tremors that the geneticist noticed were seizures.

Reflecting on her journey, Natalie still struggles with guilt. "I beat myself up every day for not just taking Cara to the emergency room," she said. "I didn't realize that what was going on was an emergency and that she was having seizures, but I knew something was going on."

The guilt is real, but what if the pediatrician had slowed down and listened to Natalie's concerns? What if that first neurologist had been less focused on getting to her next patient and more focused on Cara's symptoms? What if Natalie had simply accepted the microduplication as the full diagnosis and just went on with life? Natalie, showing resiliency and tenacity, fought hard for her daughter to get an accurate diagnosis.

When he was five years old, Rachel Bennet's son Henry was diagnosed with cortical/cerebral visual impairment (CVI), a brain-based visual impairment that is the leading cause of childhood blindness. The diagnosis came after years of false reassurance from multiple physicians that Henry would catch up with missed milestones and was "fine."

"Why didn't I go find a second opinion? Why didn't I trust my gut? Because I didn't realize at that point that the medical system isn't set up for our disabled kids. I realize that now, but it's taken ten years for

Battling Guilt Post-Diagnosis

1. Acknowledge the enormous effort in planning your child's medical care. In other words, think about everything you've done right. For instance, you've been there for your child during their treatments, you've researched and sought the best medical advice, and you've made sacrifices to ensure their well-being.

2. Remind yourself that you weren't in this alone. If you missed something, it's very likely multiple doctors, nurses, and family members did too. You are part of a team. Sometimes getting the correct diagnosis takes time and symptoms are overlooked or misdiagnosed.

3. What would you say to a friend in this situation? Try to talk to yourself the same way. It might sound like "I did the best I could with the information I had."

4. Give yourself permission to express your guilt without letting it morph into shame. It's important to understand that guilt is a feeling of responsibility for doing something with negative consequences, whereas shame is more focused on self-worth, making you feel that you're a bad person. Self-awareness can help you navigate your emotions more effectively and feel more in control.

me to get there. I now realize my kid was dismissed and I was gaslit over and over again," she said.

And as for forgiving herself for what she didn't know? Rachel told me, "I'll get there. That's what I'm working on now."

Receiving a correct diagnosis and having a clear understanding of all the factors that impact your child's disability is no easy feat. Some families fight for years to get a diagnosis that makes sense, and in turn blame themselves for missing hints that in hindsight seem so clear. But you don't know what you don't know, and it's important to be gentle on yourself as you navigate the diagnosis maze.

Violet, mom to Oliver, found the missing piece of her puzzle when her son was diagnosed with Kleefstra syndrome at the age of thirteen. Receiving the diagnosis had an enormous impact on their lives and ability to understand Oliver's needs. Early in Oliver's life, Violet noticed he was different from other kids his age. Still, she kept hitting dead ends when it came to a diagnosis. In 2009, as Oliver's behavioral issues escalated, Violet reached a breaking point.

"We felt broken. His behavior had become so toxic, we needed help. Our family was imploding," Violet said.

This is when a geneticist finally offered whole exome sequencing, a new form of genetic testing. Four months later, the results came back.

Recalling the moment when she learned of Oliver's diagnosis, Violet said, "I was driving home and received a phone call from the doctor with the diagnosis. I was floored. I had to pull over. I was so happy to have an answer. We already knew that whatever it was, it was going to be profound."

"For us," she continued, "getting the diagnosis was a relief. We spent months researching and reading as much as possible. Finally, things started to make sense. Through the diagnosis, I've also been able to connect to other parents of kids with Kleefstra syndrome, which has been the biggest help of all."

Still Looking for Answers

Maybe you're reading this and finding yourself longing for a diagnosis. Many children with chronic medical issues and disabilities have no obvious answer, which can make caretakers feel completely alone in their parenting journey.

This exact experience is what brought John into my therapy office. John had a three-year-old daughter who had myriad diagnoses with no clear root cause. Her doctors had no case studies or models to help them understand how to treat her condition. A doctor might suggest a medication or make a referral to someone else, but John often felt like he was running in circles. He spent many sessions discussing his sense of being overwhelmed because he and his wife were basically navigating uncharted territory by parenting a child with an unknown condition. He explained that he felt envious of people who had kids with more common and well-known conditions. Their path might not be easy, but at least there were people who had walked down it. To John, being in this rare situation meant being alone.

Over time, John and his wife connected to other parents of kids with undiagnosed health conditions. He joined Facebook groups and started to find some common ground with other parents. He found podcast episodes about parenting kids with undiagnosed conditions and began to feel less alone. He still longed to find a clear answer that could guide his daughter's treatment, but finding a community of relatable parents was a big step in the right direction.

In the same way that a diagnosis gives a doctor a blueprint, it also gives insurance companies a reason to cover services. Chantelle, mom to six-year-old Owen, had spent her son's entire life advocating for insurance to pay for proper treatment, testing, and therapies. Owen was nonspeaking and unable to walk, self-feed, or use the bathroom by himself. He relied on Chantelle for everything.

"Undiagnosed may not sound bad, but undiagnosed is not something that qualifies for services. It's almost impossible to get insurance to cover services for Owen. We're completely drowning in medical debt," Chantelle said.

Like any other parent, Chantelle was desperately searching for an answer that would help connect the dots for her son. She did what any parent would do: She paid for testing and treatments out of her own pocket. It's easy to see how flawed our system is when you see how a six-year-old with as many struggles as Owen is denied treatment.

"It breaks my heart over and over to not find answers. Sometimes it feels like a waste of time, but I must try," Chantelle said as she reflected on advocating for her son.

Advocating for an Undiagnosed Child

These tips come from Anne McKenzie Brendel, a lawyer and mother to a child with an ultrarare diagnosis. Anne has spent much of her time researching and working alongside specialists to find her child's diagnosis.

- Find a developmental pediatrician for your child. They are the key to connecting you to the right therapy teams and other providers.

- If your child is under three, see if they qualify for early intervention services. The services are free and will help with motor function, speech, eating, behavior, and more. You don't need a diagnosis and the diagnosis likely won't change the need for therapeutic interventions. After a child reaches three years of age, the public school system's special education programming steps in to evaluate and assist with therapies.

- Join online communities (such as Facebook groups like the Rare Disease Awareness Group, Parents of Children with Rare Conditions, and Parents of Undiagnosed Children). Here you can search for specific gene variants and ask if others have the same symptoms.

- Keep searching. Don't rely on your doctors to put the pieces together. Read medical journals and find the hospitals or clinics that specialize in your child's symptoms and reach out to them.

- If your child has had genetic testing, enter their genetic variants into a database, like MyGene2, to find others with the same variants.

- Prioritize seeing specialists and get a second opinion if a diagnosis doesn't feel right. Ask your pediatrician for a referral if you need one for insurance coverage.

- Ask your doctor about diagnostic research and clinical trials. You also can do your own search online for clinical trials that your child may be eligible for.

Dealing with Grief

The moment of diagnosis is like a rock thrown into a lake. There's the giant splash and we're completely knocked off our feet. Everything feels chaotic and we're trying to make sense of the new life we've been handed. Then come the ripples. At first the ripples are close together and the grief feels overwhelming, and maybe even constant. Over time, the ripples start to spread out—but they're still there, and sometimes they hit when we least expect them.

Ambiguous grief is a term coined by marriage and family therapist Pauline Boss, whose work focuses on the experience of caring for a person with dementia. Ambiguous grief highlights a loss that has no clear closure, and is a common feeling among parents of disabled children. Some of us grieve not having the experiences we expected. We grieve what our child never gets to experience. We grieve the inaccessible world around us and the fact that making meaningful systemic change feels like herding cats.

I want to be clear that you can grieve your child's experience, their struggles, the inaccessible world they live in, and the ways in which your relationship is different from what you imagined and still love every aspect of your child. You can have moments of wondering what an in-depth conversation with your child would be like or what occupation they might be drawn to if they were able to work. All these details help us feel close to people and better understand their identity. There are parts of my son I'll never get to know. There are experiences we'll never get to have together. There are beautiful parts of life that Asher will never be able to fully experience due to his disability. My guess is that the same may be true for your child too. And that, my friend, is worth grieving.

Grief can feel like a million little hidden land mines. There are obvious triggers, like watching your child experience an invasive and painful medical procedure. And then there are the unexpected ones. Something as simple as watching children pop bubbles in the neighborhood square could stir up your grief as you imagine what life could have been like if your child were able to participate. I remember a former client crying in my office as she explained how she never once got to pick out her four-year-old daughter's shoes because a physical therapist simply told her what pair would be most supportive and accommodating for orthotics. Grief is always present, and it hides in unexpected places and hits when we least expect it.

"It's the big grief," said mom Rachel Bennet. "It's the trauma of almost losing your kid. It's the trauma of seeing him in pain. But it's also the little grief of going to back-to-school night and hearing the other parents talk about their fourth graders. There are days when I feel like I'm trying to breathe on Jupiter."

In other words, we grieve the obvious losses: maybe a shortened lifespan, watching your child suffer from painful medical procedures, and lack of accessibility. But we also grieve the more subtle losses unique to our child's situation and their support needs: having a different type of relationship than we imagined with our child, realizing that our child will never be able to tie their own shoes or wash their own hair, or longing to hear our child talk about their day.

The Physical Sensations of Grief

When you first receive your child's diagnosis, you may notice a constant feeling of grief. Grief can be a physical feeling; some people describe it as a pit in their stomach or a weight on their chest. Grief may make you feel lethargic, as if the smallest task is insurmountable. Many people experience a change in their appetite. When you are grieving, food may feel like the ultimate comfort, or you might feel like you can't keep anything down. When you notice grief presenting itself this way, it's important to be self-compassionate. Make sure you're getting some nutrition in your body and trying to pursue some sort of gentle movement. Most importantly, connect with your support system and try to battle the temptation to struggle in isolation.

When your child has high support needs, your role as parent is that of forever caretaker. Your child, like mine, may be limited in their ability to communicate or engage in the activities you once envisioned taking place. I find myself often feeling disconnected from Asher because he's not able to tell me about his day or his friendships in in-depth ways. Because he has high support needs, I am often focused on his safety and helping him get to where he needs to be, and therefore less focused on connecting emotionally.

I like to remind clients (and myself) that an important part of feeling our way through grief is doing just that: feeling. We live in a culture that is all about "good vibes only" and keeping things positive. But what about when you're truly suffering? When you notice yourself feeling grief, acknowledge it. Literally say to yourself, "That's grief I'm feeling." Give it space to breathe, because the more you try to push it down, the bigger it gets. Acknowledging your grief, though it may feel overwhelming at first, is one of the first steps toward accepting that in many ways, the trajectory of your child's diagnosis is out of your control. In the same way that skyscrapers are designed to sway ever so slightly in the wind, accepting the reality of your child's diagnosis allows you to adapt to life's changes. When you're stuck in denial or avoidance, all your energy is spent resisting your emotions, but acceptance allows you to feel, process, and ultimately integrate your emotions into your sense of self. Accepting your emotions (as opposed to avoiding or ignoring them) is a key part of self-compassion.

Dealing with Toxic Positivity

After getting Asher's diagnosis, I noticed everyone was quick to offer comforting words. It always came from a good place, but often the underlying message was that people didn't want to hear about my sadness or that the whole thing just made them uncomfortable.

"You and Will are the perfect parents for Asher."

"Asher's going to exceed everyone's expectations—everything is going to be okay!"

And my personal favorite—as well as the one that always seemed to make me want to scream—brought religion into the equation: "God won't give you more than you can handle."

All these niceties send a very clear message: You can do this, and it's not as bad as it feels. But in the wake of a life-changing diagnosis, it felt pretty damn bad, and I honestly didn't know if I could handle it. Don't get me wrong; hope is important. But after a diagnosis, parents need space to express a wide range of emotions.

I would wager a pretty penny that you've come across well-meaning people who really have no idea how to effectively express their encouragement in a way that helps. Toxic positivity is the pressure to express only positive emotions, and for some reason, our culture is overflowing with toxic positivity.

Walk with me, just for a moment, down the path of toxic positivity. What comes up for you when you read the following?

"You are so strong!"

"All kids struggle with something. He'll grow out of it!"

"At least you have a child" (at least, at least, at least!).

"Everything happens for a reason."

"God gives special kids to special parents!"

Should I go on? Or have you thrown this book into the corner already? Most people just don't know what to say to us, so they fall back on clichés that make them feel better. But there's something so horribly invalidating about hearing someone say "They'll grow out of it!" when "it" is a missing chromosome or lifelong disability. These are the moments when I feel like screaming, "I have to face the reality of this, so you do too!" But most of the time, I just smile and say, "Yes, he's doing really well, isn't he?"

What is so uncomfortable about admitting the truth? Why is it so hard to say, "This is really effing hard and I wish I could make it better"?

Some people are just so uncomfortable with unpleasant feelings that they'll say anything to try to evoke good vibes only. If you find yourself conversing with a good-vibes-only person, remind yourself that that's their problem, not yours. Some people feel a responsibility to fix or ease our sadness, but that's nearly impossible to do. Sadness is a normal part of the human experience, as normal as the occasional cough. If someone started coughing, you wouldn't turn to them and panic and immediately shove a cough drop down their throat—you'd let them cough! Let's treat emotions the same way. There is a Gaelic expression, *tá brón orm*, which translates into "sadness is upon me." I love this manner of framing sadness; it's so different from the typical English "I am sad." Sadness may visit repeatedly, but it doesn't have to define us and it doesn't have to last forever.

Wishing for the Magic Button

"I would change everything if I could and make her well," said Deonna Wade. This is the piece that so many of us are afraid to admit. When speaking about our child's disability, we often feel pressure to add a disclaimer. "I wouldn't change a thing."

But the reality is that many of us would give anything to remove our child's struggles. Deonna would give anything to see Allie run again. I'd give anything to have a deep conversation with Asher or watch him play a sport he loves. These feelings of longing for a different way of life don't make us bad parents. We feel shame because we're afraid people will translate "I wish things were different" into "I don't love my child." That's simply not the correct translation.

If there was a magic button that, if pushed, would allow my son to miraculously form the missing piece of his fifteenth chromosome, I'd push that button faster than you could say Prader-Willi syndrome. Aaaaaaand (big *and*), if I pushed that magic button, would I lose parts of my son that I absolutely adore? (Yes!) Would fundamental parts of his personality change? (Again, yes!) And can I, with complete confidence, say that one version of Asher is better than the other? (Big no!)

Our children's disabilities are part of what makes them who they are. Having a disabled family member has helped my other children be more attuned to differences and diversity. It's taught them to be mindful of accessibility and to look out for other people. Asher is funny, playful, loving, and the best emailer in the city of Chicago. Removing Asher's disability could take away so much of the joy that makes him who he is.

However, I'm sticking with my initial claim. Asher's disability causes him to feel constant hunger and be racked with perseveration and anxiety. He's often dysregulated and has severe apraxia of speech and is frequently misunderstood. I wish he didn't struggle in these ways. I wish he could speak clearly and navigate the world more safely. Maybe it's a silly thought to spend time on, but I guess when it's all said and done, I'd still push the button.

But then again, maybe it's not actually our child who needs to change. My child's disability makes his life harder, but I wonder how that experience would differ if the world was more accessible for disabled people. Taylor, who has a daughter with Rett syndrome, reflected on how an inaccessible world has impacted her experience of grief.

"There's been grief about my life not looking like I thought it should. But as I've moved away from that, I've started to wonder if that life was really what I wanted. I really think the grief is more about the choice being taken away from me because I feel like my hands have been tied. But at some point, there has become a peace. Grief always creeps up, but the initial grief is gone," Taylor said.

Taylor and her husband, Ben, want to be clear that they do not grieve the child they have. They grieve the inaccessible world that surrounds their family.

"It's not my kid or the fact that I have only one kid that makes me sad," Taylor continued. "It's the lack of supportive community. When you're with the right people, the grief is more bearable. It's hard because we're in a world that wasn't designed to support disability. My grief is more about that."

And here is where it's important to point out that our children may not feel grief or sadness about being disabled. They very well may not experience grief about being disabled, and they may not feel like they're missing out on experiences. As parents, we set the tone for how our kids view themselves, which is more evidence that we must do the work of understanding how our parenting experience has impacted us. It's important that we model self-love and disability pride for our children before they internalize society's ableism.

Francisco Torres is an adult living with cerebral palsy. He offered his thoughts on navigating a new diagnosis: "When parents receive their child's diagnosis, it's completely normal to feel a range of emotions, including worry, grief, and sadness. This is because they are stepping into a completely unfamiliar territory." But as time passes, these feelings can coexist with moments of celebration. Francisco emphasized, "A parent has every right to celebrate their child in their entirety, including their disability."

If you're not to the point of celebrating your child's disability, it's okay. I have days where I feel accepting of Prader-Willi syndrome and days where I resent it with all my being. I cannot underestimate the profound impact Asher's syndrome has had on both my life and his, and I'll never know what life would be like without PWS. Celebrating your child's disabilities looks like acknowledging the good days, holding compassion for yourself and your child on the hard days, and honoring the journey you're on. Remember, the emotions you're feeling now will ebb and flow over time, and the process of acceptance takes time. It's vital to celebrate your child exactly as they are, and their disability is an integral part of their identity.

In a culture that avoids painful emotions, how do we feel our emotions without the hard stuff overtaking us? Well, thankfully, we aren't the first people to experience difficult situations, and we can learn from the wisdom of those who have gone before us. The antidote to toxic positivity lies in the ability to admit when things are hard and to avoid the urge to put a positive spin on something that is just difficult. Viktor Frankl, a psychologist and one of my favorite authors, was a Holocaust survivor and believed that his ability to withstand the trauma of a concentration camp came from his hope of seeing his family again. In his 1946 book *Man's Search for Meaning* he coined the term *tragic optimism*, which he defined as the ability to maintain hope and find meaning in life, despite its inescapable pain, loss, and suffering. Tragic optimism allows space for hardship while also looking for hope and goodness in life.

We can apply the concept of tragic optimism to our journey too. We are allowed to openly admit when and how we're struggling, all while maintaining gratitude for our child. This kind of thinking is often referred to as "both/and," meaning that multiple things can be true at that same time. For example, I love my child unconditionally, and there are many days when parenting takes an enormous toll on me. Both/and thinking encourages us to step away from black-and-white thinking and allow space for the gray in all of it.

The Shame Cycle

Oftentimes the shame cycle goes like this:

You feel a twinge of grief and think, "I wish my child wasn't disabled."

Then another part of you chimes in, saying, "Don't think that! Your child is amazing just as they are. Think of the kids who have it worse, or even the kids with terminal diagnoses!"

From there, you push the grief down, feeling ashamed that you ever felt that way to begin with.

It's easy to get stuck in the shame cycle and never really give yourself space to feel your grief. But when you notice yourself feeling grief or wishing things were different, you can instead talk to yourself the way you'd talk to a friend. Try something like "This is not how I expected parenting to be, and it's so hard to see my child struggling. It makes sense that I feel this way." When you speak to yourself with compassion, you make room for all feelings without judgment, ultimately removing the thought that you are a bad person for having natural, human feelings.

The practice of radical acceptance goes hand in hand with both/ and thinking. Radical acceptance can be characterized as the practice of accepting without judgment situations that are beyond our control and the thoughts and emotions they evoke. It emerged from dialectical behavioral therapy (DBT), a form of therapy that is often used to treat people who experience emotions very strongly, especially people diagnosed with borderline personality disorder. I love applying the concept of radical acceptance to the parenting experience because it provides us with a framework for acknowledging and sitting with hard emotions. When it feels like the entire world is encouraging us to see only the positive side of things, we deserve a reminder that it's okay and appropriate to feel more difficult emotions.

Therapist Laura Wrzesinski frequently uses DBT and radical acceptance with her clients. "Radical acceptance is a practice that comes from Buddhism and has been adapted for therapy. When we practice radical acceptance, we are making a conscious decision to accept the parts of our life that are not in our control," Laura explained.

For parents of disabled children, accepting what's out of your control is both complex and healing. You may have read that and thought, "I'll never be able to accept what's out of my control!" (I often feel that too!) But accepting your reality doesn't mean you're acquiescing, giving up, or even liking things as they are. Liking things as they are is not the goal of radical acceptance. You can dread or even hate the current reality and still accept that it is indeed your current reality. And in that acceptance, there's a sense of relief, a glimmer of hope that things can be managed.

"Radical acceptance is an ongoing practice, not a 'one-and-done' tool. You can practice it when you're having significant stressors (your child is back in the hospital) or minor stressors (you're stuck in traffic and late to a doctor's appointment). It's a tool that empowers you, giving you the control to manage even the most challenging situations," Laura said.

Let's walk through a typical scenario where we can practice radical acceptance. You're running late for an important doctor's appointment. Traffic slows to a crawl, and you realize there is an accident ahead. Instantly, you begin to feel anxiety and stress. You may find yourself bargaining with this reality by frantically looking up other routes, driving more impulsively and risking an accident, or simply just panicking in your mind about how unfair it is that you waited months for this medical appointment, and now you might miss your chance to meet with this provider.

Let's pause and practice radical acceptance. You can start by saying to yourself, "There is traffic, and I am not going to be on time for my appointment." To truly practice radical acceptance, you allow yourself to feel whatever emotions come up. Maybe you feel anger, shame, and frustration. Those feelings all make sense. It's okay to feel these emotions. Next, to practice accepting the situation, you can ask yourself,

"Now what?" To calm your emotions, you might practice some steadying breathing exercises. Then, instead of convincing yourself you can still get there on time, you might decide to phone the doctor's office to let them know you are running late. You can then turn on some music to distract from your stressful thoughts. Regardless of your choice, you can make one that honors your emotions and lets you move toward regulation mindfully.

It's crucial to give yourself permission to feel it all. Be patient with yourself; your feelings won't hurt you, but ignoring them will take a toll.

Reflection Exercise

In this chapter, we've explored receiving your child's diagnosis and the common emotions surrounding that process. However, we live in a culture that avoids unpleasant feelings, which means we often criticize ourselves for what we feel. Take a few moments to examine your emotions around your child's diagnosis (or lack thereof) and practice self-compassion in the process.

- Begin by acknowledging where you are in the process of getting a diagnosis for your child. Perhaps they were diagnosed years ago, or maybe you're still searching for a diagnosis that fits.

- What emotions come up when you consider your child's unique journey to getting a diagnosis? Do you feel:
  - *Guilt for not recognizing something sooner?*
  - *Anger or frustration at the medical system?*
  - *Hurt for the harsh way the diagnosis may have been presented to you?*
  - *Hopelessness as you try to find a diagnosis?*
  - *Grief for the journey you've been on?*

- What emotion are you most likely to judge? Can you come up with a mantra for yourself to practice self-compassion? For example, if you find yourself being critical anytime you feel grief, you could say, "I can feel grief and love at the same time."

- Consider the skills shared in this chapter (self-compassion, both/and thinking, and radical acceptance). What skill seems the most accessible to you? Can you think of a time in the future when you might utilize one of these skills?

CHAPTER 3

Making Friends with the Medical System

R eading "Welcome to Holland" by Emily Perl Kingsley is a rite of passage for parents of disabled children. The message of this brief essay resonates with many parents. In it, Kingsley describes parenthood as a trip to Italy where—whoops—the plane accidently lands in Holland. No, it's not where we were planning on going, but if we stop and look around—tulips! windmills! gently rolling hills!—we'll notice the beauty of the country. We'll discover that Holland isn't all that bad.

This essay has become a bit of an anthem for some parents; it's helped many people see their experience from a different perspective. On the flip side, many disabled people (and parents of disabled kids) find this essay patronizing. It presents disability in simplistic ways, omitting the nuances and humanity in disability.

From the purgatory I found myself stuck in after receiving Asher's diagnosis, I remember finding Kingsley's words ridiculous.

Prior to having Asher, I loved the idea of Italy. I registered for all the things I'd need there. I didn't pack a feeding tube, or a refrigerator lock, or books on estate planning for my trip. When I suddenly found myself in Holland, I wanted to love it, I really did. All my friends who had made it to Italy encouraged me to love Holland. They'd sit there at the Colosseum clinking their Negronis and twirling pasta, saying, "Ciao, bella! You got this! Why don't you go check out those beautiful tulips!" But I didn't want to see the tulips. I wanted to twirl pasta at the Colosseum, dammit, and I didn't want to feel badly about it. That's what I wanted.

A key part of your new life in "Holland" is navigating the medical system you've been newly thrown into. We've discussed the difficulty of getting a diagnosis, but what about after the diagnosis? Life moves on, medical issues continue, and once again, we find ourselves in a waiting room with *Finding Nemo* playing on repeat. Some of us enter parenthood with rose-colored glasses, assuming that the medical system will answer all of our questions. Of course, we very quickly realize that is just not the case. My relationships with doctors remind me of a slightly volatile and codependent romantic relationship; my partner (or in this case, the doctor) doesn't always listen to my needs, they often have all the power, I'm always working around their schedule, they're hard to reach, and they always keep me waiting. But when it's good and I feel like I have their full attention, my life is dramatically improved.

So, how can parents of disabled kids learn to have a healthier relationship with the medical system? It starts with stepping into our power. Parents of disabled children may not all have medical degrees, but we are the experts when it comes to our particular child. It also helps to acknowledge the sometimes painful imbalance of power between doctor and patient—and that is doubly true if you are a member of a marginalized community and have a history of distrusting doctors who dismiss or minimize your concerns. And then there is learning to navigate within the limitations of the medical system and accessing the care that exists, while still fighting for your child.

Desensitized Doctors; Shocked Parents

I remember the first time I heard a doctor utter the words *Prader-Willi syndrome*. It was Asher's third day of life, right before he got transferred to the NICU. A doctor walked into our room and explained that Asher might have PWS.

"Babies with Prader-Willi syndrome tend to have low muscle tone and show very little interest in food," she began. "But sometime later in childhood, these kids become hungry all the time. Parents often have to lock the refrigerator because the child will seek food—really anything remotely edible, even dog food or trash, and can eat until the point of stomach rupture. They're often overweight and have cognitive delays and behavioral issues. It can be a very difficult syndrome to live with." She stared at us, waiting for confirmation that we understood.

When I really reflect on this experience, I ask myself whether there was a less painful way she could have explained Asher's diagnosis to me. The truth is, the syndrome is pretty scary on paper, and nothing she said was untrue. But maybe what was missing was a sense of hope. At that moment, I needed to hear that my (and my son's) life wasn't doomed. I needed to know that there were options for treatments and therapies (all of which is true!) and that there was support out there for us.

• • •

We cannot discuss the quality of medical care in the United States without acknowledging the many ways in which doctors' hands are tied when it comes to treating disabled people. And most in the United

States are overworked and limited by the constraints of what insurance will cover. Most physicians were given very little training on specific rare diagnoses and aren't adequately equipped to treat them in a comprehensive way. This reality points to the need for self-advocacy, something that many parents haven't quite mastered.

Over and over, in my therapy practice as well as in my interactions with parents, I hear that the most harmful thing a doctor can do is dismiss the wisdom of a parent. We know our child, we know their medical history, we remember the procedures that have gone smoothly and the ones that have been a disaster. We are constantly keeping track of our child's needs and trying to make sense of the complex situations that arise. It's from these experiences that we glean our wisdom and understanding of our child's diagnosis, and when a doctor refuses to take the time to hear us out, that dismissal can lead to disaster.

Savannah is a mom to a disabled son; she is also a nurse and sits on two family advisory boards as well as the ICU committee for a hospital. By all accounts, she is a respected and experienced medical professional and mom. Her son, Jude, has a complicated diagnosis stemming from an unbalanced chromosomal translocation. Jude was scheduled to have three surgeries on his jaw with the goal of moving his bottom jaw forward to create more airway volume. Prior to the first surgery, Savannah and Jude's team of specialists agreed that it would be most effective to place a central line during surgery while Jude was already under anesthesia. His condition means that he has very small blood vessels and a history of blowing IVs (when the vein ruptures and leaks blood), so a central line would be a more reliable way to provide him with pain medication.

The morning of the surgery, Savannah was ready to reinforce the plan and advocate for Jude to have the central line. She spoke her case, giving all the necessary background to the anesthesiologist, who was unfamiliar with Jude.

"She was opposed to placing the line even after hearing the list of specialists who thought it would be beneficial and after hearing Jude's history of poorly keeping PIVs [peripheral IVs]. I should have pushed more, but instead I asked her to at least place a minimum of two peripheral IVs if she would not do a central line. She pretty much blew off the conversation, went through her normal pre-op questions, and left the room," said Savannah as she reflected on the surgery.

When Savannah entered the recovery room and set her eyes on her five-year-old son, she noticed that he had only one peripheral IV in a poorly placed location on his arm. Within hours, Savannah's biggest fear came true: His PIV blew. He was on a ventilator, just two hours out from an operation in which he had had his jaw sawed in half in two places, without sedation or pain management. He was overwhelmed with pain, and the nurses attempted to reinsert his IV more than twenty times within the next four hours.

"I was sobbing. I jumped into nurse mode, trying to find any vein of value to try and get medication into my child," Savannah said.

Finally, another nurse took charge. He didn't leave Jude's side until an IV was placed.

The implications were dire. Jude coded (went into cardiac arrest) five days later while being extubated due to the amount of sedation

You're Still the Boss

Anytime your child is admitted to the hospital, empower yourself to ask questions, even if they seem silly. Early on, I felt like I was being annoying if I was too vocal with the nurses or physicians, but over time, I learned that caring for a hospitalized child should be a collaborative venture. Doctors and medical professionals can make mistakes or miss things, so remember that it's helpful for you to be part of the care team. You can ask to see your child's chart, which will help you stay informed. You know your child best, so it's your responsibility and commitment to express your thoughts and concerns.

medications that were necessary after playing catch-up all week. Six days after surgery, Jude had a central line placed.

"After he coded and in the tumultuous weeks that followed, I really struggled with the guilt of not pushing harder for that central line in pre-op," Savannah said. "My opinion and knowledge of my son's history were discarded. I was just another overbearing mother in pre-op."

Jude had two subsequent surgeries on his jaw, just months after the first, but with different anesthesiologists, not the one from the first surgery. This time, Savannah insisted on a minimum of two IVs or a central line. In both cases, her wishes were honored, and the surgeries went much more smoothly.

"I think about everything that happened that day and it blows my mind," Savannah said. "Not only am I a veteran parent of a medically complex child, but I am also a nurse, and I had the backing of my son's specialists behind me. It shouldn't have been that way even if I was none of those things. I'm the parent. I'm the expert of my child."

Painful experiences such as these lead to mistrust of the medical system. They remind us that we must be crystal clear with our wishes. But just like Savannah, we're afraid to look like the pushy parent. Many of us, especially those of us who are women, were raised to be accommodating and go with the flow. Arguing with a doctor can feel against our very nature. But we must remember that there's a difference

Facing the Decision to Deny a Medical Procedure

If you're unsure about a medication or procedure, listening to your gut is essential. Go into appointments prepared, confident, and open-minded. The best way to prepare for an appointment is to research. Ask about the potential side effects and risks of treatments. If you're still not aligned with your provider, seek other opinions. Don't be afraid to bring all your questions to the doctor. You know your child best, and you must support and understand the treatment that is being provided.

between arguing and being direct. If you don't agree with what a physician is suggesting, ask for a second opinion. If you need to delay a procedure because your gut is telling you to do so, give yourself permission to listen to your intuition.

Medical Mistrust

As is the case with all relationships, some of us come into our relationship with the medical system with baggage—trust issues, if you will. We know that certain races and ethnicities historically have been mistreated and abused at the hands of medical providers.

Even with her expertise in family medicine, Dr. Alisha Bennet sometimes finds the medical system confusing and frustrating to navigate. She also has fears for the future when her son with autism is older and physicians begin to treat him differently. "There are so many extra things that I worry about as the mother of a Black male, but to have a Black son with special needs is terrifying. I fear what it will be like when he is not so cute and cuddly and is a six-foot 'intimidating' Black man," Alisha said.

Grace is mom to Dylan, a twenty-three-year-old man who has autism with complex communication needs as well as epilepsy. Throughout her parenting journey, Grace, a Black woman, has often felt dismissed by providers and other people within her son's support network. She's been spoken to in a condescending manner and dismissed or altogether ignored, and she has, at times, been given less information about her son's condition and treatment options compared to white parents in similar situations.

"My status as a Black woman has made my experiences navigating my son's education, health, and other needed services a never-ending battle," she noted. "I have been dismissed as exaggerating or demanding 'too much' for his immediate needs. These nonsensical thoughts motivate me to persistently stand up for him and his rights. I have to do this for my son to get services, proper medical attention, and the

Skeptical Optimism

Clinical psychologist Corinn Elmore encourages Black parents to keep a mindset of "skeptical optimism," especially when working with a provider you don't know or fully trust. She encourages you to be open to the recommendations of providers, but also to test those recommendations against your own knowledge about your child. As always, you know your child best, so don't discount your own expertise.

"If you don't agree with a recommendation, voice your concerns," Dr. Elmore said. She also encourages Black parents to do their research and consult with other trusted parents.

education that he is entitled to. If not, we will only get a Band-Aid, which is only temporary."

She went on to say, "Within society, Black women are [described] as angry, pushy, and forceful. These negative stereotypes and biases significantly impact my life and lead to adverse outcomes like micro-aggressions, discrimination in the workplace, or systemic barriers that limit opportunities and require Black women like me to work harder to achieve the same recognition and success as our peers. Having a child with a disability adds to this intersecting identity. In the world of parenting a child with a disability, being a Black woman and mother has been complex."

The catch-22 here is that it is not uncommon for parents to become angry, pushy, or even borderline forceful to advocate for their child. All the stereotypes that Grace mentioned can cause providers, consciously or unconsciously, to dismiss Black women. This is not only unjust but unethical.

Black women are three times more likely to die in childbirth than white women, so skepticism of the medical system starts before a baby is even born. Add a life-changing diagnosis to the mix and it can be difficult to trust the people who are supposed to be helping you.

The Baffled Physician

When a child has a diagnosis that occurs in just 1 in 50,000 (or more) people, it's a very real possibility that the doctor will be unfamiliar with that specific diagnosis. This is when we hope that the doctor will go above and beyond and do research and consult with colleagues. We are desperate for answers, but sometimes there is no clear answer. Often, finding answers is like walking through a corn maze. We hit a wall and turn, hoping for a clear path. There's no guidebook, there's no help. We're just hoping for the right person to cross our path, one who just might know the way out. The unfortunate truth is that sometimes physicians are right there next to us in the corn maze, which just highlights our isolation even more. The experience of meeting with a doctor and feeling like they don't get it can leave parents feeling hopeless.

Darya reflected on how working with an inexperienced provider

The Fight for Resources

Hannah Mira is autistic, has ADHD, and has a disabled son. She remembers the powerful experience that motivated her to switch occupations from teacher to therapist: "I was sitting in the waiting room while my child was doing OT [occupational therapy]. A young mom was sitting next to me with three kids. She was reading a book called *IEP for Dummies* and holding a Spanish-to-English dictionary. I kept thinking, 'This is bullshit. I want to help. This mother should not have to work this hard to get what her children need.'"

Hannah, having been through the arduous journey of advocating for her own child and for herself, understands the toll advocacy can take. She emphasizes that no one else will fight for your child like you will. It's a relentless battle, a full-time job that leaves you exhausted. The mere thought of having to fight for something as basic as a wheelchair is disheartening. It's a reality that shouldn't be a part of a parent's life, but unfortunately, it is.

taught her how to advocate for her daughter, Zahra, who has Schaaf-Yang syndrome. Darya trusted her daughter's physical therapist when she suggested that Darya order a new stroller for Zahra. But the physical therapist admitted that she had never ordered this type of equipment before, and the adaptive stroller she recommended ended up being a poor fit for Zahra.

"As new parents, we were unaware that insurance typically pays for a seating device only once every five years. So, when we tried a few months later to get an activity chair for home use so that she at least had one proper positioning seat, insurance immediately denied it, claiming it wasn't medically necessary," Darya said.

Darya refused to give up. She got letters of support and documentation of need from multiple doctors, and eventually her insurance company approved an activity chair that was a perfect fit. "I have a picture of her in the chair for the first time, and she smiled, which she rarely graces us with. I can't imagine denying a toddler any device that allows them to engage with their family or friends, but that chair changed everything for us," Darya observed.

This experience was an education on how and when to advocate for her child. "I assumed all her specialists knew best all the time and took their word as gospel," she said. "I trusted them because I was new to this world and my child needed help with things I didn't know anything about. But I felt my intuition getting louder as time went on, and now I feel comfortable pushing back on medical professionals, when necessary."

Darya perfectly summed up the learning trajectory of the new parent to a disabled child. Looking back at myself in the early days, I have deep compassion for the twenty-six-year-old version of me who was a new mom, afraid, and desperate for answers. I wish I could hold her hand and whisper in her ear, "Push for more tests, and don't be afraid to speak up and share your fears," because in hindsight, that's exactly what I needed to hear. Maybe you need to hear it too. Likewise, some parents might need to hear something like "You don't have to agree to that procedure. It's okay to say no!" The bottom line is that patients—and their parents—need the space and confidence to use their voice to seek competent and compassionate medical care.

Proximity to Care

For some parents, the biggest barrier to finding competent care is simply the distance between the hospital and their home. Some families live in rural areas and may be hours away from providers equipped to meet their child's needs. I experienced this firsthand when I was spending a weekend at my parents' house in rural Michigan and Asher had his first seizure. He was fifteen months old.

As soon as I realized he was having a seizure, I called 911. An ambulance came and transported him to the closest hospital. While in triage, I met with a doctor and tried to explain Asher's syndrome in detail, hoping that he would understand the complexities. The doctor

---

Bringing Your Concerns to the Physician

Pediatrician, mother, and my sister-in-law, Dr. Margaret Atkins, encourages parents to be direct with their provider if they feel like their questions aren't being answered. Don't be afraid to say, "I'm worried about [X], and we haven't addressed that yet. How would we check that? Is there a reason you do or do not think that's what's going on? What should I be watching for if this were a problem?" Suppose the provider is still not addressing the specific question. In that case, you can ask for a referral to a particular specialist who might be able to address the issue more effectively. At the same time, it's essential to be willing to listen and understand why the doctor isn't aligned with you. The parent is the expert on their child, and the doctor has taken thousands of hours of educational classes over the years. Ideally, it's a genuine team effort.

walked out of the curtained area and went straight to a computer. I saw a search engine pop up on his screen. He quickly typed "PRADER-WILLI SYNDROME."

My stomach sank. *You've got to be kidding me.*

I want to be careful not to imply that physicians in rural areas are incompetent or not experienced, because I'm certain that's not the case. It's just that the likelihood of any doctor knowing a rare syndrome well decreases when the diversity and quantity of their patients is low.

With as much fear as I felt in the moment, I've been able to feel a bit of gratitude in hindsight. At least this doctor had the dignity and integrity to quickly educate himself on the syndrome. I think more prideful people would have made assumptions and just bulldozed me. I'm grateful he took the time to learn about the syndrome. That moment has stuck with me forever, though, and let's just say I'm very thankful to live in a large city where doctors with all different kinds of expertise are plentiful.

Jessica lives three hours away from her son Harrison's medical team, and that team is an essential part of his well-being. Harrison has several diagnoses, including mast cell activation syndrome, epilepsy, hyperinsulinism, and intestinal failure.

"We do not have any qualified hospitals or doctors around to care for him. If something is wrong, it's a long trek to get any kind of care. I can't tell you how many times I've found myself speeding down the freeway with a vomiting, screaming, or seizing child. It's terrifying," Jessica said.

One of the scariest things about living far away from the hospital is that Jessica can't always predict how long it will take for her to get to the hospital. "Traffic is a huge factor," she noted. "Several times it's taken six to nine hours just to get home because of traffic. It causes a lot of panic. What if traffic is horrible but he needs help right now?"

There are many reasons why someone would prefer to live in a rural area, including family support, jobs, and reduced cost of living. As much as we wish we could mold our lives around our child's disability, it's just not always an option. We often have to make decisions based on everyone's needs, not just those of our disabled child.

When asked how she stays prepared for an emergency, Jessica pointed to the need for constant hypervigilance: "Always be prepared. Carry a hospital bag with you at all times because you never know when you may need it. Maintain the vehicle and always have gas. If it hits half a tank, I fill it up. Always being packed eases the stress of emergencies."

Her words are yet another reminder that the responsibility of keeping our disabled children safe can feel like a pressure cooker. Many of us have no choice but to be hypervigilant, especially if our child has high support needs. If you live far from the hospital, pack a small bag and throw it in the trunk of your car. Be sure to include a change of clothes for you and your child, a cozy blanket, fresh socks and underwear, and a toothbrush and toothpaste. Think of it the same way you think about that fresh change of clothes in your child's cubby at school. Hopefully you won't need it. But if you do, it's there waiting for you.

Isabella and her husband were overjoyed when they purchased their dream house in the country. "When we found out we were expecting our son, we couldn't stop talking about our lives there, watching him grow up. Raising him in the country on our own piece of land, with a slower pace of life, was a dream," Isabella said.

And then came the biggest surprise of her life. Emmett was born with a rare genetic condition called TARP syndrome. He wasn't diagnosed until he was two but had medical needs that required hospital stays and even emergency situations where they needed to get to the hospital—and fast.

"The first year was filled with more hospital visits and admissions than I can count," Isabella remembered, "including two instances that required an ambulance. Calling 911 and having to wait for EMS to get to us was absolutely terrifying."

Isabella and her husband were faced with a very difficult decision and ultimately decided to sell their dream home in the country and

When to Take a Break from Therapies

Pediatric therapies are sometimes one of the few actionable things we can do to feel like we're helping our child, but we must approach them with a healthy mindset. It's essential to resist the urge to over-therapize our children, such as scheduling back-to-back therapy sessions or pushing them beyond their limits. We must also ensure that we have set appropriate therapy goals.

Speech pathologist Allison Urbanus encourages parents to avoid seeing therapy as a "cure" and to find a neurodiversity-affirming therapist. "It's not about 'fixing' your child but about empowering them. The goal of therapy is to equip them with as many tools as possible to thrive in a society that wasn't necessarily designed with disabled people in mind," Allison said.

Every step forward in therapy, no matter how small, is a reason to celebrate. These small victories are the building blocks of your child's progress, and they should be acknowledged and celebrated. But it's important to also be on the lookout for signs that your child might need a break.

"It's important to remember that sometimes kids need breaks too! As a parent, it's your responsibility to recognize when your child needs a break and to take the necessary steps to ensure their well-being," Allison noted.

move closer to the city. "Being forty minutes away from his appointment locations, the conveniences of the city, and most importantly our families felt so isolating. We just knew in our hearts that wasn't a sustainable way of living moving forward. Emmett needed to be closer to his providers, and we all needed the support of our families," she said.

While the move was full of grief, there was a surprising silver lining to the move: "We didn't realize how much trauma that house held for us," Isabella said. "We lived some of the scariest and darkest times of our lives there. So while leaving that home and dream behind was so sad for us, it also allowed us to leave behind some of the trauma that was tied to that house and begin to heal as a family."

The common thread in both Isabella's and Jessica's stories is that you've got to do what is best for your family. There's no scientific calculation on the optimal distance to live from your child's medical providers. The right decision is the one that serves your family's unique needs best. This is yet another reminder that there is no blueprint to your parenting journey. There are commonalities that unite us, but ultimately, each of our paths are different.

Feeling of Powerlessness

Powerlessness is a familiar emotion for parents navigating the medical system because there are so many moving parts that are out of our control. When the system that is supposed to be our lifeline instead becomes a maze full of obstacles, it can feel maddening. I have an advanced degree, English is my first language, I have health insurance, and I still find the system frustrating. Imagine the frustration of people who aren't in such a privileged position.

To combat powerlessness, we must strive for empowerment. It's important to remind ourselves that speaking up is not just acceptable but often necessary. In the past, I've been hesitant and kept my concerns to myself, afraid to come across as too pushy or annoying. Maggie Kuhn and, later, Ruth Bader Ginsburg are both credited for saying, "Speak your mind, even if your voice shakes." That's a motto I've held on to when feeling intimidated. Remember that while the doctor has a degree in medicine, you have lived experience in parenting your child. The provider is your teammate and must be open to collaboration. Self-advocacy is not just a right but a powerful tool in navigating the medical system.

To be ready for a meaningful conversation with a provider, take three steps: prepare, regulate yourself, and speak. Preparation is key for engaging in a productive conversation with a health care provider.

Approach the discussion with a calm mind (take a deep breath and avoid letting anger dominate the conversation!). If the provider consistently dismisses you or your child's concerns or is unwilling to take your feedback, it may be time to find a new provider. This can be challenging, especially when choices are limited, but finding a provider who's a good fit is worth it. You don't have to settle for a provider who isn't meeting your needs (read that again!).

Working with a compassionate, effective provider makes all the difference, both for the child and the parent, so if a provider isn't meeting your child's needs, keep searching! But before you give up, communicate your needs and expectations and go in with the mindset that the provider is your teammate. It's been said that raising a child takes

Being Assertive When It Doesn't Come Naturally

Speaking up with a provider can feel intimidating. Here are a few tips to help you find your voice.

- Use "I" statements. For example, instead of saying "You always ignore my concerns," say "I felt dismissed after sharing my concerns." "I" statements can help the provider feel less defensive and help you take ownership of your emotions.

- Write out what you want to say ahead of time. You can use bullet points, write in sentence form, or make flash cards—do whatever helps you feel organized.

- Tell a friend or partner about your intentions beforehand so they can help hold you accountable afterward. Knowing someone will check in with you later will motivate you to be assertive.

- Avoid the perfectionist trap! Your communication doesn't have to be perfect. When in doubt, just start speaking up about your concerns. You don't have to be polished. Do your best to connect to your emotions and say how you feel.

a village, but raising a disabled child takes a village, a hospital, a pharmacy, specialized therapists, and a whole lot more. Don't go at it alone, and remember to find your community.

Reflection Exercise

Take a few moments to reflect on your strengths and weaknesses when it comes to navigating the medical system. Some of us are naturally good communicators, while others are great with organization, and still others are pros at negotiating with providers and insurance companies.

Circle the options that best describe you. If you have a partner, ask them to complete the exercise too.

STRENGTHS	
Communicating with providers	Scheduling appointments
Running and comparing numbers on bills	Organizing paperwork
Calling the insurance company with appeals or issues	Researching providers
Sitting with your child at the hospital	Communicating your needs to others
(other)	(other)

WEAKNESSES	
Communicating with providers	Scheduling appointments
Running and comparing numbers on bills	Organizing paperwork
Calling the insurance company with appeals or issues	Researching providers
Sitting with your child at the hospital	Communicating your needs to others
(other)	(other)

For the weaknesses you circled, complete the following exercise to better understand why it's hard for you and what you can do to improve in this area. See my own exercise below.

Skill: Calling the insurance company with appeals or issues

What's hard about it: I'm afraid I won't know what I'm talking about, the insurance employee will somehow make me feel stupid, and it will just be a waste of time.

The thing I dread the most about it: It's going to take so much time and I won't accomplish anything.

Someone I know who is good at this skill: My friend Ally (she always seems to figure these things out).

What makes this person good at it: She seems confident, and if she doesn't know the answer, she just asks anyway.

One small step I can take to start improving in this area: Write down my questions and concerns as bullet points so I feel more prepared for the phone conversation.

2

Kid Meets World

CHAPTER 4

Letting Go Without Falling Apart

From the moment a child is born, we do everything in our power to keep them safe—and for the parent of disabled child, that is no minor feat. We become attuned to the slightest sign of sickness and acutely understand our child's nonverbal cues—ah, the art of predicting a crisis! It's a skill that many of us have mastered. Our ability to read our child's cues and intuitively tune in to their needs is often a key part of their survival.

And then, slowly over time, we're expected to just let go.

It starts with sending our child to school or to a childcare provider. We try our hardest to trust someone else to care for our child and hope that they will give us their personal cell phone number in case of an emergency. The story plays out in many different versions, but one way or another, we all get here. Before we know it, preschool turns into high school and potty training turns into puberty, and as parents, our asses get kicked over and over by the perennial grief of parenting a disabled child. That is, our experience looks and feels so different from everyone else's and yet we're navigating a microcosm of "normal life." Everyone sends their kid to school, everyone feels the rupture of independence, everyone reaches a point where they don't know what their kid is doing every moment of the day. But the reality is, many disabled children are dependent on caretakers and adults to help them—maybe forever. The concept of independence is an unreachable myth that many of our children will never really be able to obtain, even when their bodies grow and, suddenly, we no longer see a small child in front of us but rather someone who resembles a grown adult.

When our child has high support needs, we (or another caretaker) may, quite literally, be responsible for keeping our child alive on a daily basis. We're not talking about an after-school babysitter who drives our child to ballet. Our kids often need help using the bathroom, getting dressed, eating, bathing—all of it. We are terrified of our child falling through the cracks but also desperate for the support and structure that the outside world can offer. Sending our children out into the wild and watching them grow up can be both deeply rewarding and painful, but there's no escaping it.

As our child grows and transitions into new life phases, we're evolving right alongside them. The process of slowly letting go and witnessing our child experience life outside the safety of our wings can stir up a whole lot of emotions. The first time I watched the yellow bus drive away with Asher, I felt grief because I knew he wouldn't be able to explain his day to me when he got home. It's been many years since that first day of school, and I don't feel grief when his bus drives off anymore. Now, I'm grieving his experience of being a teenager and how it's vastly different from that of his peers. Talking to nondisabled teenagers has many times caused me to go home and shed tears, realizing, again and again, the limitations of what Asher and I can talk about and how we connect. Our child changes, we change, and our emotions change too.

Watching our child become more independent can also bring us an immense amount of joy. For the past two summers, Asher has spent a week at a sleepaway camp. The camp is close, just an hour and a half away, and is specifically for kids with disabilities. Each camper has their own dedicated counselor, and the counselors get a chance to become friends with their campers and learn more about disabilities. Asher feels so proud of himself for being brave enough to leave home and make new friends. This summer, Asher was especially enthralled by the shaving cream station, where he got covered from head to toe in shaving cream. This earned him the "messiest camper" award. From my perspective, he's becoming more open to new textures and experiences, and I've never been prouder of my kid making a mess.

The truth is, everything changes when a disabled child morphs from a little kid into a teenager and then into an adult. It's easy to get worn down by the increasing physical demands, like having to lift a 120-pound child. It's easy to become exhausted by the intricacies and effort of helping our child navigate peer relationships or school. Our children change, if not intellectually and emotionally, then certainly physically. We can either grow with them or cling to the past. Either way, life is moving on.

As I write this chapter, I'm mindful that your definition of independence is probably influenced by your child's specific disability. Independence can mean many different things and is highly contingent on your child's level of support needs. As you read this chapter, consider both the areas where you feel sadness and the areas where you feel pride when it comes to your child's independence. Try to challenge what you once thought independence would look like (maybe college, marriage, living independently, and having children). Offer yourself compassion for the thoughts that cause you pain and celebrate the ways in which you've watched your child grow.

Learning to Trust

Holidays can be complicated for caretakers of people with Prader-Willi syndrome. Holidays and food are often synonymous, and unfortunately, Asher's early years at school often included food-filled holiday celebrations. One year, as Christmas was nearing, it felt like I received an email every day from the teacher asking if Asher could have more food at school. The emails often asked innocent questions like, could Asher participate in the cookie decorating contest, or have popcorn while watching *Rudolph the Red-Nosed Reindeer*?

One email read "He seems hungry this afternoon, is it okay if Asher has extra cookies at the music party today?" My eyes reread the email, making sure I hadn't misunderstood it.

I felt the rage bubbling up in my throat. Once again, I was forced to choose between being a rigid, disciplined mom by prioritizing my son's nutritional needs or a carefree, flexible mom, making room for unexpected holiday cheer.

The teacher and I had discussed Asher's syndrome in depth, multiple times. I took a moment to catch my breath and reminded myself that not feeding a hungry child is counterintuitive for most people. I was able to hold two truths at one time: The teacher wanted to make sure that her student didn't go home hungry, and she clearly didn't have a full understanding of Prader-Willi syndrome.

Primary and Secondary Emotions

Psychologist Robert Plutchik coined the terms *primary emotions* and *secondary emotions*. A primary emotion is our initial, unanalyzed response to an experience. A secondary emotion is the feeling that comes later, and it's usually a feeling about a feeling. Anger can be either a primary or a secondary emotion, but it's usually secondary. In other words, anger is often a reaction to a more immediate primal feeling.

This simple mistake showed how the most notable part of Asher's syndrome was difficult to fully grasp. He felt hungry *all the time*. Any adult in his life needed to understand this basic fact about Prader-Willi syndrome, or else his safety was compromised. The rage I was feeling was at the surface. But at my core was a deep feeling of vulnerability and a reminder that I was entrusting complete strangers to care for the child I'd built my entire world around keeping safe.

I also felt profound worry. I feared that Asher's basic needs related to his disability were unknown and that, ultimately, he wasn't safe at school. Home, on the other hand, was safe for my son. I understood his needs and was able to communicate with him. I believed his teachers and therapists had his best interest in mind, but my child was so complex. I'd known him for his entire life. How could I expect a person with a roomful of kids to be perfectly attuned to his unique needs and understand the complexities of his syndrome?

I did my best not to let anger get the best of me that day. I responded to the teacher's email taking a kind, yet confident tone. I thanked her for taking the time to send this email, but unfortunately Asher couldn't have extra cookies at the party. I went on to include yet another explanation of Prader-Willi syndrome and thanked her for understanding. I cried that day as I closed my laptop after sending the email. Not necessarily out of anger or frustration, but because I began to realize exactly how hard it would be to entrust the world with my disabled son.

The Frustrating Fight for Resources

While our experiences differ depending on our child's diagnosis, there is one common factor that nearly every parent of a disabled child is familiar with: advocacy. We've all heard about (maybe even experienced) horror stories related to IEPs and advocacy for specific needs at school. If there is one thing that stirs up emotions, it's the complexity of advocating for your child at school.

Maria's son Levi was a typically developing two-and-a-half-year-old until it was discovered that he had an intestinal volvulus (twisted intestine). The volvulus led to a devastating cardiac arrest event that ultimately left Levi with hypoxic-ischemic encephalopathy (HIE), cerebral palsy, and short bowel syndrome. In just a few moments, Levi's life was turned upside down—and so was Maria's. She went from pushing her baby in a swing to pushing him in a wheelchair. Ultimately, Levi needed a colostomy, a gastrostomy tube, therapies, a gait trainer, and a communication device.

It's been ten years since that life-changing event, and Maria continues to advocate for her son's needs. At school, Levi requires behavioral and medical support. Additionally, she has navigated classroom placement issues as well as communication and transportation issues.

She recalls a specific time she had to battle with the school for a behavioral plan. Levi would often gag to the point of vomiting, and some staff members wondered if this was an intentional behavior or a medical issue. Regardless of cause, the frequent vomiting negatively impacted Levi's health and nutrition. Maria spent a year and a half advocating for her son, going back and forth with the school, until the school moved him to a different class and ultimately brought in a behavioral interventionist to help with the issue.

In reflecting on how she managed the situation, Maria admitted that she struggles to balance kindness with assertiveness. "I feel anxious about how to approach each situation and have to tread lightly with my concerns so as not to come across [as] too forceful or direct. I still have to make my point and advocate for Levi," she said.

Many parents feel this pull. There is a part of each of us that wants to go into the school and scream at anyone who will listen. Wouldn't it feel so good, just for a moment? However, we know that very quickly that emotional release would turn into shame, and then perhaps a ride in a police car and many other issues. So, we continue to put that thought away.

One alternative is to organize your thoughts and practice a

"compliment sandwich," meaning that you give feedback in a positive-negative-positive pattern. For example, "I really appreciate the emails you've been sending, but it would be helpful if you could add more detail about my daughter's eating habits each day. I really do appreciate you giving this attention. I know you are juggling a lot."

Strategic communication with school staff is an enormous mental load to carry around. Maria also admits that the constant advocacy wears on her. "Sometimes it's really hard to keep following up on the issues and exhausting to keep being the squeaky wheel when I already have so many other things on my plate," she said. But Maria never forgets her "why": "With his condition, I feel that he's trapped in his own body sometimes. I know he is trying to communicate his needs and if I can't help him do that then I am failing him."

Dealing with Stares and Whispers

Ever since Asher was little, eating out at a restaurant has been complicated for our family. Portions tend to be much too large, even when we order from the kids' menu. We usually try to sneak half of Asher's french fries off his plate or swap a chicken tender for fruit without him noticing. This was much easier when he was younger. Regardless, venturing out to a restaurant almost guarantees that there will be some sort of food-related meltdown. We've just grown to accept it. However, these meltdowns were much less disruptive when Asher was a baby. Onlookers might assume that he was late for a nap or just a fussy baby. When a sixteen-year-old cries and jumps up and down in public, it really creates a scene, let me tell you. In those moments, I can feel the glares and stares burn through me and find myself wanting to scream, "Didn't anyone teach you it's not nice to stare?!!"

But let's be honest, it's a lot less cute when a teenager has a meltdown.

I'm always struck by the complex emotions that bombard me anytime Asher struggles under the watchful gaze of strangers. My brain freaks out, but in all the wrong ways. I feel intense shame and perceive judgment from everyone around me. I assume they're thinking, "Why can't that mom control her son?" or, even worse, "What's wrong with that kid?"

I'm embarrassed to say that I (more times than not) jump into action in a performative sense to try to prove that I'm a good mom and astonished by my child's unusual behavior. I then go into fight-or-flight mode, with my main goal being getting out of whatever godforsaken place we're in. What stops me from extending compassion to my son, squatting to meet him on the floor, looking him in the eyes, and stroking his hair? Why is it so difficult to forget about the staring strangers and direct my attention toward helping my son self-regulate and calm his body? If I'm being honest, I'm often more concerned with how I look as a mom than with my son's well-being. Of course, once I'm home

How to Self-Regulate in Stressful Moments

When you're feeling activated by your child's behavior in public, pay attention to what's going on in your body. Take a deep breath and be aware of your tendency to panic. Take a moment to relax your shoulders and slow your breathing. If you're trying to exhibit calm behavior, it helps to have a calm body! Your job is to remain calm, maintain your child's safety, and try to help them regulate. It's tempting to focus on everyone else and their reaction to your child, but at this moment, they really don't matter.

Make sure that you and your child are both physically safe. If your child is on the floor, get down at their level and speak calmly. It can help to talk about what's next on the schedule and to validate how they're feeling. Try something like "I know you're angry right now. Let's take a deep breath and think about what movie we're going to watch when we get home."

The least helpful thing you can do is to engage in a power struggle, shame your child, or lash out.

and able to calm down, I slip into a guilt and shame cycle, struggling with the very questions I'm asking myself here.

I'd venture to say I'm not alone in this behavior. In these moments of heightened stress, we must tap into our ability to self-regulate. When I have been able to offer a gentle smile to a stranger and get one in return while my teenage son is crying, I feel empowered and even encouraged by the people around me. Nine times out of ten, onlookers wish they could do something to help. Very rarely are they judging or scoffing at us (although I'm sure it happens occasionally). Next time you notice yourself feeling emotionally flooded due to your child's behavior in public, take a beat to regulate yourself. Remind yourself that your job is to keep your child safe, and you're not responsible for everyone else's reaction. Try to hold compassion for your child (and yourself!) and remember that a meltdown does not indicate bad parenting.

It's important to point out the difference between my child's response and my response in these stressful situations. I have the power to shape how Asher views himself and whether he feels shame in the aftermath of a public meltdown. As parents, we need to remember that we set the tone for how our children view their disability long before anyone else has the chance to do so. Our responses matter greatly.

It's not just a disabled child's behaviors that can garner unwanted stares; it's physical differences too. You'd think that as a civilization we would have learned by now not to stare at people, but as it turns out, that's just not the case.

Matthew, dad to Fiona, age ten, has noticed a change in how people look at his daughter as she gets older. Fiona has a noticeable facial difference: a large vascular birthmark that covers half of her face and body. "As she's grown older and is out in public, the blatant stares have become disturbing. It's a distressing experience for her, and I can feel the weight of it," Matthew shared.

Matthew and his family recently stopped to use the bathroom on a road trip. Fiona was immediately uncomfortable because so many people were staring at her, and Matthew noticed it too. "There's a noticeable difference as she's grown older. It's natural for people to smile at a baby or toddler, but it seems like people are less conscious of their reactions now that she's maturing," he stated.

This unwanted public attention is, of course, experienced by wheelchair users, people with physical differences, and anyone who might have a noticeable disability. Seeing your child gawked at, especially by adults who should know better, is infuriating. My son doesn't have noticeable physical differences, but I can imagine that if he did and strangers were staring at him, I would want to scream and point out everyone's bad behavior. But as parents, we set the tone. It's helpful to have an arsenal of responses and be able to manage your personal feelings in the moment. The first step to navigating unwanted attention directed at your child is to, *when possible*, get their consent on how you respond.

Matthew and his daughter have formed a strong bond in managing unwanted stares by working together as a team. It always starts with acknowledging how Fiona is feeling. "I can usually tell when she's feeling uncomfortable, and I'll ask her if she wants to leave whatever space we're in. After we leave, I'll ask her what she's feeling and allow her to talk about it," Matthew said.

When all else fails and the stares are just excessive, Matthew and Fiona use humor. "We recently were in Target," Matthew recalled, "and this woman turned her head and gawked at Fiona. Fiona and I looked at each other and started laughing. Afterward, we joked about all the funny things we could have said to the woman. It felt cathartic to say to each other, 'Take a picture; it lasts longer,' and poke fun at the woman's lack of self-awareness."

Sometimes people's curiosity gets the best of them, and they'll actually approach Fiona. More times than not, people direct their questions to Matthew ("What is on her face?" or "What happened to her?"). Matthew will then turn to Fiona and say something like "Do you

Giving Your Child Space to Feel

Fiona, a ten-year-old with a visible facial difference, has always felt supported by her parents. She believes that the most validating thing a parent can do is allow their child to experience and express all emotions about their disability or difference.

Fiona said, "Sometimes I just want to be like everyone else and not have a birthmark. But I also know that my birthmark is important to me and makes me stand out. There are times when I feel like if my birthmark disappeared, I would be sad."

As parents, it's crucial to create a safe space for our children to express their feelings about their disabilities, but don't assume their emotions are all heavy! As Fiona pointed out, her birthmark is an important part of who she is. When your child is struggling with their disability, it's natural to want to shield them from painful emotions. Still, just as we allow ourselves to feel the full spectrum of emotions in our role as parents, we should also encourage our children to respond to their disabilities honestly.

feel comfortable talking about this right now?" This simple question empowers her to share her medical information as she sees fit, respecting her autonomy and needs.

Reflecting on his emotional response to his daughter being stared at in public due to her birthmark, Matthew said, "It makes me feel angry more than anything. I empathize with my daughter and feel sad if she feels sad, but more than anything, I just feel angry that people don't know how to function as normal human beings. I don't expect people to say we don't see differences. Of course, people will notice someone with a facial birthmark. But is it too much to expect grown adults to recognize that staring makes people uncomfortable? It's just common sense."

Our Kids; Other Kids

As hard as we try, we cannot always protect our children from the pains of social interactions. Even events that are happy and celebratory can feel laced with sadness if your child is struggling with friendships—a sentiment that every parent can related to regardless of disability status. But for the parent of a disabled child, there can be an added layer of complexity. I often find myself struggling when Asher is misunderstood in social settings or not able to take part in conversations because he doesn't fully understand what's being talked about. There are also just many experiences he's not able to participate in. Anything involving strenuous exercise or certain coordination skills will be difficult for Asher. It's easy for me to experience feelings of being left out by these missed opportunities, even if that's not how he is experiencing them.

Vanessa watched her son Jordan play on the Special Olympics basketball team. He is tall (really tall), at well over 6 foot 5 inches. He also was born with hydrocephalus, a condition that impacts his verbal and cognitive abilities. Vanessa reflected on the sting that occurred in a moment when she should have been happy: "It's a weird juxtaposition. Everybody comes—all the 'regular' kids come to support your 'special' kid. And they feel like they're great people because they showed up to one game and made a sign. But then they never invite Jordan out to go to coffee."

We want our kids to be more than someone else's good deed. We want our kids to be included—really included, not in a way that is placating or infantilizing. Adolescence is a time of meaningful development in friendships, and the reality is that sometimes our kids get left behind. Whether our child struggles with verbal expression or low cognition, teenage friendships move forward, and our kids can slip through the cracks.

Vanessa went on to discuss her own anger: "You sit in this gym where all these kids are trying so hard. On one hand you should feel grateful, but it just makes you feel the opposite. It just makes you feel mad. These games are inclusive, and I should be happy, but I just find myself feeling so mad."

These feelings spill over to friendships in general, especially for high-achieving parents who care (maybe a little too much) about their image. (I'm raising my hand here; it's me.) I often find myself feeling worried that Asher's friends will eventually fade away because he struggles with maintaining a conversation. For example, Asher loves video chats with his nondisabled friends (mostly girls), but he's not cognitively able to have in-depth conversations. These discussions often last just a few minutes, and they are fueled solely by the friend's ability to engage Asher, not the other way around. Lately, Asher pulls up "The Friday Song" by Rebecca Black on YouTube and plays it for whoever he's talking with. This is very Asher. Routine, predictable, comforting.

Knowing When to Step Back

Ashley Harris Whaley is a disabled activist and founder of Disability Reframed. She reflected on how her parents empowered her and fostered self-confidence while she was growing up. "They were always very good at striking a balance between never overestimating me and never underestimating me," she said. "They were always very in tune with my capabilities and limitations."

Regarding independence, Ashely highlighted the difference between advocating for kids and teaching them to advocate for themselves, if possible. "My parents did a good job of knowing when to pull to the forefront of advocacy and when to take a step back and teach a man to fish. They understood that I could handle it. You must know your kid," Ashley said.

Most importantly, Ashley always knew her worth, which was empowering: "My parents never apologized for me. They never made me feel like I had to shrink myself, which is an experience that the world demands of disabled people daily. The world wants us to take up less space and make it so that everyone else feels comfortable. My parents never played into that."

I sometimes worry his friends will get annoyed, and deep down inside I worry that they're doing a good deed and not actually interested in a friendship with my son.

I never want Asher to feel like a burden to anyone, especially a well-meaning teenager. Inside of me is some tangled combination of wanting to protect Asher, wanting to protect myself, and fear of burdening someone else. We've all seen the pictures blasted on social media of a kindhearted person who gets all the credit for taking a disabled classmate to prom. That good deed turns them into a hero, and the subtext on these posts is that without that thoughtful kid, the poor disabled child would have sat home alone on prom night. That's not equity, that's pity. The difference between performative friendship and real friendship is in intention. I just want to yell, "Don't pretend to be my child's friend to use it as an extracurricular on your college application! Because when you reach your goal of getting into college and suddenly no longer need a friendship with my son, guess who's going to be left feeling lonely and sad? That'd be my kid, not you."

Keeping Our Kids Safe Online

One day not too long ago, I was mindlessly scrolling Facebook when I noticed a familiar face in my suggested friends list—Asher Atkins. I didn't even realize that Asher had Facebook, and now the algorithm is suggesting him as my friend? I had some questions. How did he sign up for Facebook? Who are his friends online? And most importantly, what is his online behavior and is he safe? Navigating internet usage for all kids is complicated, but especially so for vulnerable kids with varying degrees of cognitive abilities. it can be even harder to protect them from the dangers lurking on the internet.

Matthew, dad to Fiona, reflected on his feelings about his daughter being online: "The thought of bullying and social media scares me. I'm terrified of when my daughter opens herself up to any criticism from people at school or strangers on the internet. I feel really scared

Staying Safe Online

Internet Matters is an excellent resource that can help you and your child navigate the internet in a responsible way. This non-profit organization's Inclusive Digital Safety hub was designed specifically to address issues of internet safety for disabled children. Internet Matters offers a free online course to teach caretakers how to help their disabled child use the internet in a safe way.

for her and I want to prepare her for the realities of social media. I'll shield her from it for as long as I can because no middle schooler or high schooler should have to deal with that sort of thing. Her social media will be highly filtered."

But really, how do we shelter our kids from social media in this day and age, when every kid seems to be consumed by it? This question takes us back to our fundamental struggle with independence. How do we foster independence in a world that can be unsafe for our disabled children? How do we protect them while not controlling them?

I wish there were an easy, cut-and-dried solution to the question of internet safety for disabled children, but there's not. The appropriate path for your child probably lies within your intuition. You know your child's unique abilities, vulnerabilities, support needs, social needs, and ability to understand danger. It's important to take all these factors into consideration when deciding on internet usage. Wherever you land, I want to acknowledge the potential grief in this decision and process. You'll see other people's nondisabled kids displaying their colorful, curated life online. There may be a moment where you feel the stab of jealousy and sadness that your child's life might look nothing like that. You may battle this feeling by saying you're thankful that your child isn't involved in the chaotic and dangerous world of social media, but alongside that relief is often sadness that they can't participate. It's a double-edged sword, as is the case on so many fronts of parenting, and your feelings can be a complex reflection of that paradoxical situation.

Tips for Safe Internet Usage

Foster trust and communication by implementing an open-door policy for your child's social media use. Let your child know that you'll be checking their messages and activity and do so often. Be clear that it's not okay to send or receive photos of bodies. Also, openly discuss bullying and other inappropriate online behavior. Being direct about what kinds of messages and behaviors are unsafe and unacceptable is crucial, empowering you in your role as a parent and your child as they navigate the internet.

• • •

Letting go is hard. Your child's unique journey toward independence is based on a hundred little details. Is your child influenced by their peers who are making friends, dating, or fully jumping into life in the wild? How is your child able to engage in the world around them? How dependent are they on you for day-to-day care?

And then there's you. Your identity has, of course, been shaped by the amount of time and energy you've spent caretaking for your child. For many of us, letting go isn't an option. We long for independence, but due to medical and emotional reasons, it's like walking a tightrope to balance our child's needs for independence, dependence, and interdependence.

My advice to you: Determine what independence means to you and your child. Maybe it's advocating for the perfect power wheelchair so your child can be more in control of their ability to navigate the world, teaching them how to respond to people who make them uncomfortable, or using a communication device to express themselves. Maybe independence means someday living alone, walking, or being able to express their needs and wants. Your job as the parent is to cheer your child on, honor where they can assert their own independence (no matter how big or small), and acknowledge your own shit when it comes up throughout the process.

Reflection Exercise

Regardless of your child's abilities, they have unique social needs, passions, and strengths. Take a moment to reflect on the following questions to help you better understand what independence might be like for your child and for you.

- How do you envision your child seeking independence in the future?

- What are some of your worries about the struggle for independence?

- What are your biggest fears related to independence?

- What safeguards need to be in place for your child to have a sense of independence? (Think about caretakers, resources specific to your child's diagnosis, medications, assistive devices, and so on.)

- What do you need to feel supported as your child moves toward independence?

- If your child will ultimately have very little independence from you, take a moment to write down your feelings about this. What support do you need as your child gets older and physically grows? What are your hopes for your child? What are your hopes for yourself?

CHAPTER 5

When Puberty Strikes

Each new year ushers in growth, and before we know it, our sweet little three-year-old is a middle schooler and then a high schooler. And herein lies the unique grief of being the parent of a disabled child: Our child continues to grow older, but in many ways, they never grow up. Their bodies may look like adult bodies, but depending on their cognitive and verbal abilities, the vulnerabilities we usually associate with small children may forever exist.

We entrust others to keep our children safe, but not without anxiety. How do we let go but still stay close in case something unexpected happens? How do we handle our emotions as we watch our child's classmates get driver's licenses, go on first dates, and eventually graduate from high school and move on to college, jobs, and adult lives when we feel like, in many ways, our child has been left behind? The emotional journey that runs parallel to these experiences is profound, and sprinkled in it are sadness, jealousy, guilt, and disappointment.

Navigating Our Kid's Sexuality

When I was pregnant with Asher, my mind wandered to what his life might be like once he got older. I was so excited for the teenage years. I always viewed myself as a person who was open and comfortable with sexuality, and I wanted to have a household that normalized and celebrated the human body and self-expression. I was eager to teach my son about consent and respect. I wondered: Who would he be attracted to? Would he eventually start a family and make me a grandmother? I had taken multiple college and graduate classes on human sexuality and felt like I was up for the task of raising a boy who would treat others with respect and be an overall good human.

I still hold those values close, but the way it's all played out has looked a lot different from what I expected. There have been no conversations about dating or sex yet, and though they may still come down the line, truthfully, I suspect they will not. It's hard to gauge what my son can comprehend when it comes to sexuality and romantic relationships. But just because Asher is not capable of using complex words to describe the human life cycle doesn't mean it's not important to talk about sexuality and consent in a broad way with him. He may never get married in the traditional sense, but he will (and does!) have meaningful friendships with many people. I've learned that as parents of disabled kids, we can't shy away from the topic of sexuality. Even if we stumble our way through it, we must have open communication with our children about safety and sexuality and present it in a way that they are most likely to understand.

• • •

It was Wednesday at 3 p.m. and Fatima plopped on my couch just as she had every other week for the past year. I know therapists aren't supposed to have favorite clients, but Fatima had grown to be one of mine. Her son Stephen was seventeen and had level 3 autism, which meant that he had high support needs and severe communication deficits. Fatima and I often worked on navigating what it meant to parent a disabled child. She struggled with many of the same things most parents struggle with—anxiety about the future, frustration with her son's behavior, and navigating her marriage and friendships. But on this particular Wednesday, Fatima had something urgent to discuss, and I could tell by the look of concern on her face.

"I walked in on Stephen masturbating," she blurted out.

"Wow, we're getting right to it today, aren't we?" I took a drink of my mint tea and crossed my legs.

"I shouldn't be surprised. But I mean, wow, there it was. I guess I just wasn't prepared for it," Fatima added.

We discussed her initial response, which she admitted was disgust and embarrassment.

"It's just so complicated, seeing my little boy with the body of a man," she admitted. "Of course he has hormones drowning his system just like any other boy his age. But in almost every other way he is still a toddler."

"What feels most scary about admitting Stephen has sexual urges?" I asked.

"I worry about him being taken advantage of or exposing himself in public. He just knows it feels good. He'll never be mature enough to fully understand sex—it's just an impulse. That's scary. That feels really scary," Fatima said. "I've been so focused on Stephen's behavioral stuff that I never even thought about this. I did notice a stain in his underwear a couple of times while I was doing laundry, but maybe I wasn't ready to face it yet. I was in denial, I guess."

I nodded in agreement. The thought of our disabled children growing into disabled teenagers brings with it a unique set of concerns, sexual development being just one of them.

Ultimately, Fatima was able to explain to Stephen that masturbation is something we do in private, just like going to the bathroom or showering. She also discussed pleasure, normalizing the physical response of ejaculation to reduce any shame around the act of masturbation. She did all of this in a simple and judgment-free way to open the door to discussion.

"I have never talked about masturbation so much," Fatima said.

It wasn't easy, but eventually Fatima felt like Stephen understood the boundaries around private touch and was able to demonstrate more appropriate behavior.

Much like Fatima, I struggle with the thought of my disabled son desiring sex, mostly because I'm not sure he can offer or fully understand consent. When it comes to teaching my son about sex, I have all sorts of feelings of avoidance and discomfort. The good news is that the public school system usually provides some sort of sex education, although it's difficult to say how comprehensive and helpful it is. A parent's fear is often that their child with cognitive impairments (or in special education in general) may slip through the cracks. Disabled students may attend sex ed classes with their nondisabled peers, but the material may not be easily understandable or taught in a way that is accessible. In all cases, regardless of disability status, parents must fill in the gaps and ensure that their child is empowered and comfortable with their sexuality and changing body and that they understand this complex subject in a way that is reflective of their cognitive abilities. For some students, this may be as simple as knowing what appropriate touch is, and for others it may be a more thorough explanation of masturbation, sexual touch, menstruation, and reproduction.

Periods and Pregnancy

Oh, the joys of getting your period for the first time! Menstruation is a rite of passage and brings with it a whole slew of things to worry about. First off, there's hygiene. Especially for disabled people, menstruation can spark concerns about cleanliness as well as dignity. Does your child need assistance with using period products? Who can be trusted to help with such an intimate task? With menstruation, of course, can also come the potential for pregnancy, which then brings into question all sorts of important topics such as consent, sexual assault, and communication. Menstruation and a change in hormones can also exacerbate epilepsy and other seizure disorders, as well as impact mood and mental health.

Historically, there hasn't been much information, support, or many solutions provided for disabled people who are menstruating or for their parents, and there are still plenty of barriers in this area. For starters, it's often difficult to find a public bathroom where a disabled person can comfortably take care of themselves (or be taken care of). Whether it is changing a tampon, a pad, or a menstrual cup, a disabled person may need more space than a standard toilet stall can offer. Physically, a disabled person may have difficulty inserting or removing a tampon or cup or changing a pad and may require an assistive device or another person's help. Thankfully, recent years have seen improvements in adaptive clothing, including period underwear.

Hormonal birth control is an accessible and effective solution for disabled people because it can stop menstruation and prevent pregnancy. Birth control can also offer solutions to the issues of hygiene and dignity.

Bailey, a college professor with two daughters, ran up against multiple constraints when helping her daughter Delilah care for herself while menstruating. Delilah has been diagnosed with autism and sensory issues and has always been resistant to wearing underwear. This presented a challenge when she started her period at the age of twelve.

"We had an issue at school where she tried to put a pad in her leggings and got blood all over herself. Cleaning her, how she smelled—it all was hell," Bailey said.

Because of this, Bailey and her husband made the decision to put Delilah on birth control. "She doesn't get her period anymore, which has been really helpful. If she got her period now, she wouldn't be able to go to school on those days," Bailey said.

There continues to be new and exciting developments that help disabled people and their caretakers manage menstruation in a clean and dignified way. From tampon insertion accessories to period tracking apps, new resources are popping up all the time. But this doesn't entirely take away the hardship of navigating a child's menstruation and risk of pregnancy.

Birth control can be a life-changing resource for disabled people and their caretakers. It can preserve dignity by allowing good hygiene and offering independence from reliance on other people during a vulnerable time. How you choose to help your child manage their menstruation is a deeply personal and intimate decision, of course. If you are able, include your child in this complex decision-making process, allowing as much consent and collaboration as possible.

The most common fear I hear from parents of disabled menstruating people is that they're afraid their child will be sexually abused and ultimately end up with an unwanted pregnancy. This is a terrifying thought on so many levels. Many of our children cannot offer consent or even verbally express if someone has abused them. Even in the modern day, some parents feel so desperate to avoid pregnancy that they consider the most extreme measure to prevent it.

Bodily Autonomy and Consent

The US has a long history of abusing disabled people. At the turn of the twentieth century, it was common practice for a panel of men to determine whether a specific woman was fit to procreate. If the men in power decided any given woman was unfit to have children, she could be surgically sterilized against her will. In her book *A Disability History of the United States*, Kim E. Nielsen tells the story of Alice Smith, who in the early 1900s was sterilized against her will just months before her eighteenth birthday. Alice had a documented diagnosis of epilepsy, and both of her parents had been deemed "mentally deficient." An in-depth study was done on her family, and it was eventually determined that sterilization would improve not only Alice's life but the greater society at large. This is one story out of many just like it.

Sterilization has long been used to ensure that disabled people do not procreate, which is ultimately a form of eugenics. In 1907, Indiana became the first state to allow the forced sterilizations of disabled people. In 1927, the US Supreme Court voted to legalize the forced sterilization of disabled people, which in turn made the act much more common. By 1963, more than 60,000 disabled people had been sterilized against their will. As of 2007 (not that long ago!), a disabled person's family and caregivers can meet with a physician to determine whether sterilization is best for that person. While laws have been put in place to protect disabled people, forced sterilizations are still allowed in thirty-one states and Washington, DC. In these states, a judge can determine whether to sterilize a disabled person. This is a complicated issue that can very quickly become abusive.

When, if ever, is it okay for a parent to make the decision to sterilize their child? As parents, we make all sorts of decisions for our child. For example, Asher's scoliosis was recently at a sixty-five-degree curve. We had to pursue spinal fusion or else his lung capacity would be compromised. As much as we brought him into the decision and explained what was going to happen, we ultimately made that decision for him. This is one of many examples of the type of decisions a parent might have to make for their child.

When it comes to sex and pregnancy, what happens when a person is cognitively unable to offer consent, let alone parent a child? Is it okay then to make a decision as big as sterilization for another human? Many of our disabled children are unable to offer consent, either to sex or to sterilization. Take Elissa's daughter, for example. Abby, at seventeen years old, has spinal muscular atrophy and requires round-the-clock care.

"As it stands right now, there is no way Abby could engage in a consensual sexual relationship. It terrifies me to think of that. Not because she doesn't deserve pleasure, but because cognitively she cannot offer consent. If she were to be sexually assaulted and become pregnant, we would have to terminate the pregnancy. All of that would be terrifying for her. Pregnancy alone could kill her," Elissa said.

Jennifer is mom to Margo, age fourteen, who has cerebral palsy and support needs that will require her parents to be her primary caregivers for life. Margo started her period at a very young age, and hygiene immediately became an issue. Under the guidance of a pediatric gynecologist, Margo was given a shot to suppress her menstruation. She's been receiving that shot for almost five years now, and it's not recommended that she continue using it much longer.

"In a typical scenario, I would never even think of such a permanent decision [like sterilization] for my daughter. It's heartbreaking to have to entertain this level of intense decision-making," explained Jennifer. "We have talked to her in a developmentally appropriate way about adulthood and what that may look like for her. It's one of the hardest parts of parenting a disabled child," Jennifer admitted. "She can understand what is different about her life, which can cause her sadness. But that doesn't change her future, unfortunately."

As complex as the situation is, especially for parents trying to consider what is best for their children, disability advocates, disabled people, and human rights organizations clearly state that the forced sterilization of people with disabilities is an act of violence. As parents, we must listen to these voices and find alternative solutions for preventing pregnancy (and, equally important, preventing sexual assault) for our children.

When it comes to our biggest fears, sexual abuse of our disabled child is right at the top. The reality is that disabled people are four to ten times more likely to be sexually abused than their nondisabled peers. This abuse often goes unreported because the survivors are not always able to effectively communicate. Abusers are predominantly male (although that certainly doesn't mean they can't be female) and are almost always a person whom the disabled person trusts.

This touches on separate but related issues, which is that it can be very hard (and very expensive) for disabled people to find qualified caretakers. Parents may feel like they need to just "take what they can get" to accept help, which can lead to unqualified candidates caring for their children. The staggering systemic issue is that the care of disabled people is not a priority for our society. Parents are often left with very few resources, and our kids are put at risk.

Preventing and detecting sexual abuse is nuanced and complex. You must consider your child's cognitive and communicative abilities. Does your child respond to visual prompts? If so, use flash cards to explain appropriate touch and what is off-limits. If your child can communicate, get in the habit of talking about who is allowed to see their body (for example, only the doctor and only when a parent is in the room). If they require assistance in the bathroom at school, remind them about what sort of behavior is appropriate and what is off-limits. If your child is not able to communicate or is severely cognitively impaired, these conversations become more difficult.

Like many of us, Bailey worries about her daughter being vulnerable to sexual abuse. "I worry about a neurotypical person taking advantage of Delilah. She wouldn't know how to defend herself, and she gets really worried about disappointing other people. If she had someone she trusted and they wanted to sexually assault her, she would easily be a target," Bailey said.

Educating our children empowers them to be informed and serves as a protective factor against abuse. Admitting that our children are sexual beings forces us to face difficult questions. But what if our child is coerced into sexual activity? What if our child is the perpetrator in sexual abuse? How do we discuss these topics with our children, especially when they are cognitively impaired? These topics are often seen as taboo and not talked about openly, but that is just more reason to start discussing sexuality with our disabled children.

Sasha Tweel is the former assistant director of Rape Victim Advocates (now known as Resilience) in Chicago and mom to a teenager with Prader-Willi syndrome. According to Sasha, the two most important protective factors against sexual abuse are consent and communication. However, she cautioned, "when we're talking about people with disabilities, we're talking about so many different kinds of people. We're talking about different levels of understanding and abilities to communicate, so I don't think there's a one-size-fits-all approach to preventing sexual abuse."

Sasha went on to explain that as parents, we have to do our best to ensure that our children understand consent to the best of their abilities. That effort should be interwoven into everything. If we're helping our child put on a brace, we can explain what we're doing and ask if it's okay. If we have to unbutton their pants to help them use the

How to Help Your Child Understand Consent

1. Start young. It's never too early to instill the concept of consent. Even when they're little, allow your child to choose whom they hug and when. Before Grandma goes in for a big hug, ask your child, "Do you want to hug Grandma?" It's not rude for your child to say no. If they say no, ask if they'd like to give a high five instead. This proactive approach helps your child learn to say no when they feel uncomfortable.

2. Make a point to tell your child what you're doing when it involves their body. For example, "I'm washing your back now," or "Now I'm going to change your diaper." This helps them feel included as you care for them and allows you to communicate consent.

3. Determine what resources your child enjoys most. Is it picture books? Websites? Songs? Use your child's favorite tools to explain what body parts are private, who is allowed see them, and when. This flexible approach ensures that you can adapt to your child's preferences and needs.

4. Discuss consent during doctor appointments. For example, Asher's endocrinologist examines his testicles to assess for puberty, and every time the doctor says, "I'm going to look at your testicles. Remember, this is only okay if Mom or Dad is in the room with you." It's a clear way to explain what he's doing, why, and when it's appropriate.

bathroom, we can ask first. Even if our child isn't able to verbally communicate with us, it's important to explain what we're doing and why.

Sasha acknowledged that this is not easy work. "Trying to make sure that everyone—both our children and everyone they interact with—is behaving appropriately can be a full-time job," she said.

The thought of my disabled son being sexually abused makes me feel sick. It's just another layer of complexity as he navigates the world as independently as possible because I can't be with him for every moment of the day—which, to be clear, is not something either of us wants. But I struggle with gut-wrenching thoughts, like whether my child would even know if he was being sexually abused. And I acknowledge that it would be easy to coerce him into something he didn't actually want to do. The bottom line: We must keep talking about this. The more we keep these conversations going, the more empowered our children will be.

Dating and Sex

It's important to acknowledge that most of our kids will long for romantic love and connection. It may be hard to accept that they can have such big, grown-up feelings, and the thought of our child getting their heart broken can feel overwhelming. Despite this, disabled kids get crushes, want to go out on dates, and hope to fall in love, just like everyone else. Once again, we find ourselves at the crossroads of independence and dependence, and we have to somehow, as clumsily and imperfectly as it may be, struggle through. What works for your child may not work for mine. A true handbook on navigating dating for our disabled children would be impossible to write because every child is different in their abilities, needs, cognitive abilities, and communication skills.

Carolyn's daughter Lily developed her first romantic relationship at the age of fifteen. There had been a celebration at the end of a national conference for Lily's genetic syndrome, a chance to dress up, cut loose, and have fun. It was here that Lily and Isaiah, two teenagers who shared the same syndrome, spent time together on what felt like a first date. Their tearful goodbyes were a testament to the depth of their feelings for each other. Carolyn, who had always instilled in Lily the values of consent and emotional health, welcomed this new relationship with open arms, just as she had any other aspect of Lily's life. The catch to the budding relationship was the distance—Isaiah lived in Florida, Lily in Illinois. But Carolyn reassured Lily that they could bridge this gap with a trip to Florida in December—five months away, which to two love-stricken fifteen-year-olds felt like an eternity.

Lily and Isaiah talked nearly every day in those months between visits. And, of course, Carolyn kept her promise. In mid-December, Lily's family boarded a plane and flew to meet Isaiah and his family. "It was so lovely and sweet," Carolyn remembered. "Isaiah wore a tie and had flowers for Lily. We sat with them during their dinner because they were still only fifteen. There are so many similarities between them, which are related to their syndrome and otherwise. The kids influence each other."

However, any relationship, especially between two young teenagers with big feelings and challenges, comes with risks. Like any mother, Carolyn wants her daughter to always feel loved and cherished. But, naturally, her joy is tinged with fear because she is afraid of the potential for heartbreak.

Carolyn recognizes that Lily and Isaiah's relationship is real, even though they're young. "They obviously find great comfort in one another just by being together. They laugh all the time and have a deep understanding of each other. Lily is convinced that she and Isaiah will be married someday, and I could see them cohabitating with support," Carolyn said.

• • •

I know many of you reading this have children with high support needs. The difficult reality is that your child may never go on a date with a potential romantic partner. Your focus is likely spent on your child's health and survival, and talking about sexual development is nowhere on your radar. Maybe the only thing you can fully relate to in this entire chapter is the fear of sexual abuse. Perhaps reading this chapter stirred up your grief and brought back a familiar old voice that says, "I'm not even understood here." I know that feeling; I often have that inner voice too. I encourage you to take what you need from this chapter. Your child's unique abilities have no impact on their fundamental need for safety, consent, and appropriate sexual development. The more critical point is that we must all acknowledge that our children are complex, full humans with sexual desires who need guidance on healthy development and expression. As with everything, we must meet our child where they are and determine the most appropriate way to foster healthy relationships with others and themselves.

As a parent, you play a crucial role in fostering your child's sexual development. Simple actions such as labeling your child's body parts when you're bathing them can give them language and model open communication about their body. Empower your child to let you know when something is hurting or needs care. Don't shy away from this necessary task. The conversation doesn't have to be perfect; it just has to be had.

Reflection Exercise

As parents of disabled children, we may find that the struggle to ensure our children's safety as they navigate the world independently is draining and exhausting. The stark reality is that disabled individuals face a significantly higher risk of sexual abuse than their nondisabled peers. It is our duty to empower our children with ability-appropriate information and skills to maximize their safety. To effectively support our children, we must first navigate our own emotional journey regarding their sexual development. Use the prompts below to explore your concerns, emotions, and values around addressing this topic with your child.

- Describe the grief and/or anxiety you feel when you consider your child's desires (or lack of desires) for romantic/sexual relationships in the future.

- What is your biggest fear when it comes to your child's sexual development?

- Who are the people in your support system with whom you can be open about these fears?

- If your child is already an adult, is there a specific situation related to your child's sexual safety or development that needs to be addressed?

- When you envision your child as an adult (and even if your child is an adult), what values feel most important when it comes to their sexual development? (Some examples include safety, independence, hygiene, dignity, and self-expression.)

- Set a reachable intention for yourself as a parent that reflects your answer to the preceding question. An example might be "I will always do my best to prioritize my child's dignity and safety."

CHAPTER 6

Reaching Adulthood

I remember sitting in church as a little girl and watching a family of three—two older adults and their adult disabled child. They'd often walk in late, the son and the mom linking arms. The son usually colored with crayons during the service and occasionally made unexpected noises while the pastor was speaking. It didn't seem to faze his parents, nor did it bother anyone in the church. I couldn't tell you the man's diagnosis, and as a kid, I didn't give it much thought. I just knew that every Sunday, the three of them would walk in together, three grown-ups, one of whom required a lot of care and assistance while navigating the world.

I never thought my life would resemble that family from church—that in retirement, there would be a good chance it would be "the three of us," not just my husband and me. The concept of being a forever parent is one I never really considered. As I wonder what the future will look like, there's a big, bold question mark when it comes to Asher's independence. I guess all parents could say the same, but I find myself wondering where and how Asher will live. Will he live in a residential home or with us? How will he adjust to his younger brothers moving out and starting their independent lives? Will he be able to have a job? Will he have serious health issues? And, of course, the question that haunts all parents of disabled children: What will happen if my husband and I die before my disabled son? Who will take care of him then?

The majority of adults with Prader-Willi syndrome do not live independently, although a small percentage of them can, with support. I anticipate Asher living with us until his brothers move out, and then maybe he'll want his own version of independence too. By the time his youngest brother goes to college, Asher will be twenty-five years old.

The Advocacy Never Ends

When Bianca's son Lane turned eighteen, he became eligible for social assistance from the government in Canada, where the family resides. Once the funding was approved and the bank account was created, Bianca noticed that the money wasn't being deposited. She called the social worker, who eventually determined that the money was being deposited into the wrong account because of a mistake made on the bank's end. Bianca then spent hours in a very complicated process correcting the mistake on behalf of her child.

"How on earth would my son, who cannot count, tell time, or do his hygiene without prompting, have been able to coordinate getting his money returned to him? All the while not being able to pay his rent or buy groceries because he has no income coming in?" Bianca wondered.

The advocacy never ends, whether your child is three or thirty-three. When asked what advice Bianca has for parents of younger children, she said: "Be as prepared as you can be. Talk to teachers, social workers, other parents in the same situation, or parents of disabled adults who have done the transition. And advocate. Never stop advocating."

Of course, there are so many unpredictable, uncontrollable variables involved in the future, but it's constantly on my mind. I'm not there yet, but I can see this reality on the horizon. My husband and I have established a will and a special needs trust and started taking the legal steps that will ultimately lead us to guardianship of our son once he is legally an adult.

Shifting from School to the Outside World

As we settle into high school with Asher, I'm thankful that he'll be able to stay at his current school until he's twenty-one. Most schools in the US allow children with IEPs to stay in high school until they are in their early twenties, but what happens after that? Consistently, parents of disabled adults have shared that the transition from high school to, well, whatever is next has been difficult. As parents, we go from working closely with the school system, which is filled with activities, clubs, and opportunities for our kids, to relying on the outside world to hold our families.

Vivian is the mother of two disabled adults, both in their twenties. In the absence of the structure that school once provided, she observed, she has had difficulty finding her footing: "The world no longer has space for my children to operate without me. When they were younger, there were opportunities for them to be somewhere without me. There were also places I could go without them—adult activities at church, book clubs, playing in a band. As their opportunities have diminished, I find they start coming with me everywhere and my identity disappears. This all happens just as my friends are reinventing themselves outside of being a parent."

As I reflect on this transition, I'm reminded of bringing my tiny baby home from the NICU. In some strange way, the transition away from school and into the "world" must feel eerily similar to leaving the NICU. The only difference is that our baby is now a lot older—and so are we. Think about it: What did you feel when you left the NICU? If your baby wasn't in the NICU, what did you feel in the moment when you got the diagnosis or when you realized you were now responsible for a child with a whole lot of needs? I felt panic, isolation, and a huge sense of responsibility. When our baby turns into an adult and leaves the comfort of school, we'll be forced to redefine community and find support all over again.

The Search for Resources

When Bianca's disabled son Lane transitioned out of the school system, she immediately missed the structure and resources he'd left behind. As she observed:

> Parenting a disabled child feels like a team effort. Your team is made up of a pediatrician, specialists, teachers, and multiple therapists. These experts all work alongside you to help your child. Parenting a disabled adult, on the other hand, is an independent project. You're launched into this whole new stage of life with zero support—other than the supports you seek out and put in place on your own. No one is knocking down your door to tell you how to handle all this. Our support system is small, and we now focus on developing skills to maintain the status quo. I miss getting emails from teachers giving me updates about my son and suggestions for skills we could be working on.

We know we need resources after our disabled child leaves high school, but how do we begin to find the right programs and partners? Megan Turner and Leslee Schafer found themselves asking that exact question, especially as Megan had a child who has lifelong support needs. After realizing there was a big, gaping hole in accessibility and services for adults with disabilities after high school, Megan and Leslee cofounded a nonprofit in Illinois called Our Aging Services. Megan heads up the developmental disability side of the organization, specializing in securing government resources, transition planning, and IEP support. When she's not running her nonprofit, she specializes in vocational readiness and transition planning for students aged eighteen to twenty-two in a public school in Illinois. But her number one priority is her son, Hank.

Hank is a teenager and has myriad diagnoses, including myoclonic atonic epilepsy (also known as Doose syndrome), Lennox-Gastaut syndrome, autism, and cyclic vomiting syndrome, among others. Megan has made it her life mission to help disabled young adults find community and support. As both the parent of a disabled child and an expert on support services after high school, she urges parents to plan ahead, as hard as it may feel.

"Don't count on the state servicing your child. Don't assume that everything will get taken care of if you pass away," Megan said.

"We have to normalize the conversations about the future starting at a young age," Leslee added.

"The timeline is very important," Megan continued. "Services like ours can help you access available programs or fill out paperwork. Our goal is networking, getting resources, and helping families. When you're raising a disabled child, thinking of the future is what keeps you up at night. We can't entirely take away your anxiety, but if we can ease some of your stress, we're doing our job."

Leslee noted, "Finding the time to ask for help and do what needs to be done is the hardest constraint for parents. They're so consumed with the day-to-day."

The day-to-day is often all a parent can face at any given moment, but once your disabled child hits their early teenage years, it's important that you begin to consider their options for after high school graduation. This process can be scary, and it's natural to want to avoid it. But just like with every other aspect of parenting, you have to process your emotions and keep putting one foot in front of the other. That may look like slowly putting away money to save for legal services or ensuring that you have a will or trust in place. You may begin to explore your child's options for programs after high school, or maybe your child is cognitively able to go to college and just needs some support getting there. The urge to avoid thinking about the future is understandable, but by thinking ahead, you're planning for your child's safety and easing your own anxieties too.

Facing the Hard Decisions

Ellen and Jeff had four biological children when they adopted their son David. At eight years old, David had come from a situation of extreme neglect, and Ellen and Jeff were committed to giving him a supportive and loving home.

Fast-forward to today. David is in his fifties. He has several diagnoses, including schizophrenia and a developmental disability. David lived with his mom and dad for a long time, but as he grew older, he began showing aggressive behaviors toward his family members, going so far as to physically attack one of his younger brothers. It was at this time that Ellen and Jeff made the difficult decision to find a place for David to live that was safer for everyone.

Ellen was overwhelmed with guilt after she made the decision to move David to a residential home. She felt like she was abandoning her child, even though in her heart she knew it was the safest decision for the entire family.

"I had to admit that I wasn't able to take care of my son anymore. It's so hard for a mother to face that. David is my child and I just never imagined him not living with us. But it's important to realize that there are other people out there who can offer support," Ellen said as she reflected on the emotional process of finding a new home for her son.

Ellen also can admit that David loves his independence. He watched his siblings grow up and move out of the home, and being able to do the same gave him a sense of pride. "David has his own apartment and bathroom. He was able to pick out his own shower curtain in his own color scheme—not mine. That was really important," Ellen said.

Ellen and Jeff were able to connect with helpful community resources that were invaluable in making the transition a smooth one for David, but this decision took bravery and trust. As it would for any of us who parent a disabled child. We spend our child's entire life involved in nearly every decision about them. In fact, depending on our child's abilities, we may be responsible for every single aspect of their care. Surrendering that responsibility to someone else may feel like we're losing a part of ourselves. This loss is different from sending our child to school because, for the first time in many years, we may then have the opportunity to rediscover our own identity apart from being our child's primary caretaker.

If your child is currently young, consider what it might feel like for them to be older and out of the house. You might feel a mix of emotions: anxiety, guilt, grief, relief, freedom. These are all normal and appropriate emotions to have in this experience.

As parents, many of us become so consumed with our responsibilities that we also become completely cut off from what brings us joy. There just isn't much time (or money or childcare) to allow us to pursue our own interests or hobbies. It sounds so simple, but we have to prioritize time for ourselves. I know, I know, this is so much easier said than done, and I'll be the first to admit it's not easy. The ability to foster self-care begins with giving yourself permission to do so. You have to believe (really believe) that it's important to allocate time to you. Maybe you take ten minutes of your lunch break to walk outside in the sunshine, or you download an app on your phone that makes connecting with your friends easier. Perhaps you and your partner take turns sleeping in the guest room so you're both getting a full night's sleep a couple times each week. What is it that fills your cup? What activities and nonnegotiables do you need in order to show up as a whole person each day? Begin with answering these questions and then see where you can fit in whatever form of self-care you need. Prioritize it as you would a specialist appointment for your child.

Ellen reflected on this process as she thought about what advice she would give to a younger parent. "The thing is," she said, "you cannot let parenting a disabled child consume you entirely. When David moved out, I was able to volunteer and continue to pursue my own passions. Even when David was younger, both sets of grandparents were involved with caretaking, and that allowed me to have breaks."

She continued: "Get help, get support. Find a group of people who understand, where you can vent about the things that are weighing you down and people get it. Also, it's okay to grieve, but don't think that this is the end. Your child will grow up and find their own version of independence, and it's okay to let them go. You will feel all sorts of feelings when you admit that your home might not be the best place for them anymore, but it's good for your child to have their own sense of independence. My biggest advice: This isn't something that is going to destroy your life and tie you down forever. Your life will never be the same, but this is not the end of it."

A Beginning and an End

Carla had been a client of mine for a few months. She'd never been in therapy before, but her best friend had encouraged her to find a therapist. This was an especially difficult time for Carla because Charlotte, her thirty-year-old daughter with Down syndrome, had recently moved into a residential home. Carla was a sixty-six-year-old single mother and Charlotte was her only child, so this transition was a huge adjustment for both Carla and Charlotte.

"I joined a pottery class. I'm trying not to hate it," Carla began.

We talked about her efforts to find new meaning in her life. The time that she used to spend caring for her daughter was now wide open. Carla was newly retired and suddenly found herself with a quiet home and an empty schedule.

"I know Char is happy. We talk every day, multiple times. She was bored with me at home and needed to have her own life. But I worry about her, and I miss her," Carla said.

Carla worried a lot. She struggled to trust the caretakers at the group home to be attuned to Charlotte's needs in the same way she was. Carla worried about Charlotte making friends or having to eat a meal alone. Over time, however, Carla's perspective on her relationship with her daughter shifted.

"I always just assumed that it was Charlotte who was dependent on me. My whole life was built around keeping her safe. But now that she's not living with me, I'm realizing that I need her just as much as she needed me. I depended on her for companionship, and she gave me a sense of meaning in my life," Carla said.

This realization was a huge turning point for Carla. She began to think about what she enjoyed (apparently pottery was not it) and how she could begin to pursue her own interests. A whole new world was open for Carla, even though Charlotte's newfound independence was terrifying.

Working with Carla got me thinking about how our lives become intertwined with those of our children. Most parents simply assume their child will go through natural milestones, moving toward independence. But for some of us, it's hard to believe that a day will ever come when our schedules won't be determined by our child's needs. Independence isn't the primary goal when it comes to parenting a disabled child; their survival and safety is.

Finding What Works

Kathy and her husband James have made the choice to keep their adult son Peter with them in their own home. Peter is autistic and has high support needs. Kathy and James know their son best and feel strongly that keeping him in their home for as long as possible is the right choice for everyone.

"With his receptive language being his greatest struggle, helping him understand why he isn't living with his family anymore would be almost impossible. His heart would be broken. The idea of him feeling rejected or abandoned is the most painful thought I can imagine," Kathy said.

When you're making decisions about long-term care for your adult disabled child, you're making a choice not just for now but for the sustainable future of your family and your child. Whether your child stays with you or moves elsewhere, you'll experience many complex emotions: By now, you are well acquainted with these emotions; guilt, anger, jealousy, anxiety, and grief. But amid these feelings, you may also find relief, pride, gratitude, and excitement at the chance to rediscover yourself.

We must allow ourselves the space and permission to grieve but also remember to hold onto hope. The future is hopeful. In my interviews with parents of adult disabled children, each one shared a similar sentiment when asked what advice they have for younger parents. There's so much to celebrate about having an adult disabled child; for example, their unique sense of humor, their one-of-a-kind personalities, and, most importantly, their very existence.

Kathy shared an example of her son's gentle ability to mirror the values she and her husband made a point to instill: "When Peter is calm, he is the most kind-hearted young man. When he was a little boy, I taught him to pray anytime he heard a siren. I explained that someone was in distress and praying was something we could do to help. To this day, he continues his prayers anytime he hears a siren. He has a sweet heart of gold, and I hope my husband and I had something to do with his compassion and kindness."

The Ability to Adapt

Lane, now in his mid-twenties, lives at home with his parents. He was born at twenty-five weeks of gestation, suffered a stroke when he was six weeks old, and was later diagnosed with autism. For most of Lane's life, his parents assumed he'd be able to live independently when the right time came.

"As Lane was making his way through high school, we started to work toward him living on his own. We planned on setting him up in a one-bedroom apartment nearby and popping in daily to check in," his mother Bianca said.

But shortly after his high school graduation, Lane had a seizure—his first in more than fourteen years. "I could tell almost immediately that something was off," Bianca remembered. "He seemed a bit more confused at times, more scattered. He was unable to do the things he had been doing for years, like remembering to take his medications or practice his daily hygiene. He started a small fire in the oven while making nachos—something that he had done independently every night for the past two years. We started to notice a lack in balance, strength, and coordination. His conversations became harder to follow and he just started to disengage."

Lane's family was forced to shift his goal of living independently because it no longer felt safe for him to live alone. An MRI was done to see if there was a physical reason for the regression, but the neurologist couldn't find an explanation. "We want independence for him, and he desperately wants it for himself, but at this point, the risks are greater than the reward," Bianca said.

Lane's family members pivoted in the exact way that they needed to, but the change in plans was a hard reality to face. Bianca and her family went back to the drawing board to restructure what life would look like moving forward. "As a family we are struggling with balance when it comes to caring for Lane and our younger two sons. Although Lane is twenty-two, we still have to manage him much like a young child. That is difficult when we're trying to balance his wishes and rights as an adult," Bianca said.

Bianca and her family are committed to providing a safe home for her son, but she's not giving up on the potential for his independence someday. "Lane will remain at home with us for now and maybe we can reassess if the right situation ever arises," she said.

Lane's story is a reminder that we cannot assume that our children's stories are completely written. Bianca is doing her best to remain flexible in terms of what is best for Lane. While there's grief involved in Lane's unexpected shift away from independence, his safety and well-being come before everything else. His family will continue to be a safe landing place for him, for as long as is necessary, because that's what families do.

When We're No Longer Here

One question haunts us all: Who will care for my disabled child if I'm no longer here? And how do I plan for that? This is yet another reminder that we must plan for the future with our child's well-being in mind. It's a difficult reality to face, but having a plan in place can ease a bit of our anxiety now.

Brittany remembers sitting at her stepmother Teresa's bed in the intensive care unit. Teresa had fought a hard battle with an autoimmune disorder and yet another antibiotic-resistant infection was finally winning.

The room was full of nurses and family members, as everyone knew the end was near. Brittany and her stepmother locked eyes across the room.

"Take care of my girl," Teresa whispered.

"I promise, I will," Brittany responded.

Those were the last five words Teresa spoke, and Brittany has kept her word and taken care of her stepsister, Becca, ever since.

Becca has autism with high support needs, an intellectual disability, and epilepsy. She is thirty-three years old, the same age as Brittany. Brittany is no stranger to the world of disability, as the younger of her own two children is also disabled and will likely have lifelong support needs.

Brittany's dad married Becca's mom in 2008, and the stepsisters had an instant connection. Noticing their special connection, Teresa asked Brittany if she would be willing to be Becca's guardian when Teresa passed away.

"I said yes without hesitation, assuming that her passing wouldn't be anytime soon," Brittany said.

But sadly, in 2022, Teresa became very ill. Brittany and her stepmother revisited their earlier conversations about Becca's guardianship and Brittany again promised she would take care of her stepsister. Just a few months later, Teresa died.

"I was very overwhelmed the first year. I even contemplated telling my dad I couldn't do it. I had to get a lawyer and refile for guardianship. It has been extremely stressful," Brittany said.

Before Teresa died, she legally made Brittany co-guardian of Becca. While at the time this seemed like the right thing to do, it complicated things in the long run because Teresa remained Becca's legal guardian.

"If there's one word of advice I'd give to parents," Brittany said, "it would be to legally transfer guardianship over before you get too sick to do so. My stepmom was organized, but somehow many of Becca's important documents have been misplaced. For Becca to receive Social Security benefits, I need all those documents. I can't get those documents unless I'm her legal guardian."

Becca lives in a residential home for disabled adults and has full-time caretakers. She stays with Brittany on weekends and holidays. Thankfully, this arrangement feels sustainable, partly because Brittany understood Teresa's desire to have her disabled daughter taken care of. Brittany shares that desire for her own son and recognizes the peace of mind it brings to a parent to know their child is cared for.

"When I doubt myself on the hard days, I remember my promise to my stepmom and I think about what I'll need someday. I hope I'm blessed with someone like me," Brittany said.

I hope I'm blessed with someone like Brittany someday too. In fact, most parents will tell you that their biggest fear involves who will care for their child when they're gone. This responsibility often falls on a sibling, but it's important that parents don't assume a sibling will want or be able to care for their disabled sibling. It is ultimately the parents' responsibility to ensure that there is a plan in place for after they die. This task may feel daunting and terrifying, but this is just another instance where facing our fears is worth it in the long run.

It is a gift for your disabled child to reach adulthood—and adulthood brings with it a lot of hard decisions. As caretakers, we have to navigate circumstances that no parent ever imagines having to navigate. Who will care for my adult child if I'm not here, and how will

Facing Your Fears About the Future

Let's be honest, thinking about the future can be immobilizing. It's easy to put off preparing for the future because it just feels too overwhelming. But here's the good news: Facing your feelings of anxiety and tendency to avoid is the first step toward relief. It's normal to want to avoid hard feelings, so, now, get specific about what it is you're afraid of when it comes to the future. Is it that you feel guilty because your child may need to live in a residential setting away from you? Is it anxiety about who will take care of your child when you're gone? In the words of Dr. Daniel Siegel, "Name it to tame it." The less ambiguous your fears are, the more effectively you can problem-solve.

I afford the astronomical costs associated with care? Where will my adult child find community? Similarly, where will I find community as I discover room to explore my own identity? With each answer comes a cycle of emotions: grief, guilt, anxiety, relief, freedom. None of these reactions are wrong; they're just part of being human. Meet yourself with compassion as you look toward the future, or care for yourself now as the parent of a disabled adult.

Reflection Exercise

Where Do You Find Your Sense of Self?

As your child transitions into adulthood, you may notice that you feel disconnected from yourself. Your sense of self, broadly defined, means your understanding of who you are. Your sense of self includes connection to your interests, likes and dislikes, values, and identity. So often as parents we lose our sense of self to the endless to-do lists and identity as a parent to a disabled child. But we are more than just a parent (even if "parent" defines a meaningful part of our identity). So, now, take some time to reconnect to who you are and with your interests, passions, and values.

List four values that are important to you (for example, community, faithfulness, happiness, generosity, honesty, kindness, fairness, equality, competency, justice, peace, pleasure, wisdom, religion, meaningful work, curiosity, beauty, or artistic expression).

1.

2.

3.

4.

For each value you listed, brainstorm one way in which you demonstrate that value in your everyday life.

Value 1: _____

Value 2: _____

Value 3: _____

Value 4: _____

- Is there a specific value that you'd like to be more intentional about pursuing? If so, which one?

- Can you brainstorm some activities or hobbies that might help you embody that value?

- Can you think of an activity you undertook in the last year in which you felt connected to one or more of your values?

  - *How did it feel?*

  - *When is the next time you'll be able to do this again?*

3

Taking Care of Yourself

CHAPTER 7

Facing Your Anxiety

I've always been on the anxious side. When I was young, I would worry about the safety of family members driving during a snowstorm or my mom getting a follow-up mammogram. But my anxiety became debilitating after Asher had his first seizure when he was a year old. We later found out that it was a febrile seizure provoked by a virus. After the seizure, I became hypervigilant, drawing meaning from the most minor things that might indicate a seizure was looming. I've never told anyone this before, but I noticed Asher yawning a lot the first time he had a seizure. My wise brain knew that he likely was tired from the virus that provoked the seizure, but my anxious mind grabbed on to the idea that yawning was an indicator of a seizure. I quickly convinced myself that anytime he yawned, he might be at risk for a seizure.

For parents of disabled or medically fragile children, anxiety about our children's well-being is ever present. Our minds are constantly searching for warning signs, trying to help us stay one step ahead. Many of us have experienced our child having a sudden, terrifying medical event. Our constant state of hypervigiliance leaves us unable to truly relax or be present. The persistent anxiety can lead to caregiver burnout and complete exhaustion, a reality that many of us face daily.

For me, anxiety became especially intrusive after the birth of my second son, Silas. On paper, you'd think a normative birth and postpartum experience would calm my anxiety, but I became hyperfocused on what could go wrong. While I was still in the hospital after labor, a nurse took Silas for a bath. I woke up in a panic because he hadn't been returned yet. I was convinced that he had had a seizure and the medical team had to resuscitate him.

I usually recognized that my anxiety was irrational—Silas had no signs of any health issues and no known disabilities. But just a year earlier, Asher had been admitted to the hospital for a full week because he had multiple seizures back-to-back. So, while there were no signs that my new baby was having seizures, my brain remembered the danger and was trying its best to protect me by keeping me on guard.

I was a full-time stay-at-home mom and was overcome with dread anytime my husband left for work. I felt completely terrified to be home alone with my kids, almost to the point that I couldn't function. Even if there were no signs of danger, I could not relax. I was constantly hypervigilant, checking my kids' temperatures and watching them obsessively to make sure nothing seemed "off." I even avoided going places because I was afraid something bad would happen and I wouldn't be able to handle it in public.

Apparently I'm not alone in these experiences. I polled 315 parents of disabled children, and 98 percent of them said they struggle with anxiety about their children's health. To put that another way, only 6 of the 315 parents reported not having anxiety about the health of their disabled child. If you're reading this and are among the 2 percent who don't struggle (my husband confessed to me that he responded to my poll and was indeed part of that 2 percent), please share your secret!

Our brains so desperately want to stay ahead of the trauma. Anxiety is an attempt to predict the bad thing that will happen as an act of self-protection. We think that if we spend time obsessing about what might happen, it will be less of a blow when it does happen. When I think of it from that perspective, it makes sense that many of us are racked with worry, hypervigilance, and, of course, anxiety. Most of us were completely caught off guard when something terrible happened to our child, and our brains are desperately trying to make sure we're never caught off guard again.

Kathleen knows exactly what health-related anxiety feels like. On top of being pregnant during the height of the COVID-19 pandemic (enough to put anyone on high alert), Kathleen gave birth to a son, Jameson, with a rare genetic mutation that has myriad symptoms, including immunodeficiency, seizures, and developmental delays. She didn't learn of Jameson's full genetic profile until almost a year after his birth.

"It's this invisible load that permanently sits on my chest," Kathleen admitted. "Even when we go through periods of time where there's a lull in appointments and illness, I find it incredibly difficult to relax and enjoy the moment. I'm constantly on edge, waiting for the next medical emergency to occur. Sometimes this anxiety is intertwined with sadness, anger, resentment, or even guilt. My family has come so far from the newborn days, but our story is far from typical and we are always in the trenches of medical issues."

Neurobiology 101

Our brains have one main goal: our survival. This means that our brain is always gathering information and trying to predict what's next in an effort to protect us from potential harm. If you were bitten by a dog when you were young, you may still flinch anytime you're approached by a scary-looking canine. If you got side-swiped at a certain intersection, you may always approach that intersection with caution (or even avoid it altogether).

The first time you experience a traumatic event (maybe the first time your child has a medical emergency), your brain is caught completely off guard. This frightening moment causes neurons to fire off in

Psychedelic-Assisted Therapy

There is promising new research coming out in the field of psychedelic-assisted therapy that could serve parents in processing trauma and anxiety. Therapist Staci Berman helps clients who want to discover new neural pathways and face decisions in a new way.

"In typical psychotherapy, it can take a long time for people see their circumstance in a different way. Ketamine and psychedelic therapies offer perspective in a much more concentrated way. Something chemical happens that allows for more perspective and for you to relate to your circumstances in a different way that offers new possibilities for you," Staci said.

"I try to be clear that it isn't a magic bullet," she added, "but I have seen powerful changes in ways that people might not have expected. Maybe they come in hoping things will change in this massive way, and the change turns out to be very small but very significant. Even just a slight change in thinking can totally change your perspective."

a specific sequence or pathway. Neurons are nerve cells that communicate to our muscles and basically allow us to comprehend the world around us. Think about driving your car in the grass. The first time you do it, the grass will flatten temporarily. But if day after day you drive that same path, eventually the grass will permanently flatten. Neural pathways are exactly the same. The more often the neurons on a specific pathway fire off, the stronger that neural pathway becomes and the more natural it becomes for your brain to rely on that particular response. So, if your child had a medical emergency, and you panicked and leapt into life-saving action and your child survived, your brain is going to see that as a win. The next time you perceive a similar threat, your brain is going to remember your previous experience and prompt the same response as it did before. This combination of a perceived threat plus a strong neural pathway makes for an almost automatic response. In other words, if you think your child might be having a health emergency, you freak out because that's what worked before.

Because of this, small triggers might evoke a big reaction. That path in the grass is so familiar that the thought process happens without you even realizing it. If your child is sick with a harmless cold, your brain still steps in and says, "I'll take it from here! Emergency!" Then it's off to the races, with a panicked, freaked-out reaction that would be appropriate for an emergency, but maybe not for a cold.

The Ultimate Fear

At the core of health anxiety is a deep fear of death. But for many of us, the fear of losing our child is actually not irrational. Many parents of disabled children have had experiences where we thought our child might die. Over time, carrying the weight of this enormous worry takes a toll. While most children recover from medical emergencies, far too many disabled children die young, and their parents are left behind trying to cope in a world where everything feels wrong. Being a parent with anxiety around sickness is problematic because sickness is a normal part of parenting. All kids get sick. Yet after experiencing the death (or near death) of a child, our alarm bell is broken. It can be difficult to assess if something is "normal sickness" or "emergency sickness." Everything begins to feel like an emergency and a parent tends to always carry a sense of hypervigilance around illness.

Kasey's daughter Hannah died just eleven days after her first birthday due to a severe congenital heart defect. Kasey also has an older son, and after experiencing the medical trauma and death of her daughter, she continues to struggle with health anxiety.

Kasey was forever changed by her daughter's death, but it was Hannah's life that had the biggest impact on everyone who knew her. "She lit up the room with her smile. It was infectious. She loved to snuggle and hold anyone's finger," said Kasey as she reflected on her favorite details about Hannah. "By the time she passed, her hair was just starting to come in enough for her to have two little dirty-blonde pigtails. She had chubby little cheeks and was the sweetest, most perfect little angel.

"Now that my daughter has passed, my heart races when my son gets so much as a cough. It helps for me to call a doctor's office for the smallest of questions. If everything is truly fine, I'd at least have the reassurance that I said something. My daughter's diagnosis allowed me to become an excellent advocate, something I was never really good at before," Kasey said, reflecting on how she manages her health anxiety in the aftermath of losing her daughter.

Why Pop Psychology Coping Skills Don't Work for Us

When I'm in the throes of anxiety, I try to remember that I'm a therapist. I do this for a living. Shouldn't I be able to help myself? Why is this so hard? In those moments, I think back to every client I've worked with who struggled with anxiety and wonder if they felt like my little tips and tricks were just bullshit. Deep breathing? *But I feel like I can't breathe at all!* Exercise? *There's no way I could focus on anything except my anxiety at this moment.* Count to ten slowly? *This feels like an emergency! There's no time to count to ten!*

I often feel like most of the well-known coping skills proffered by pop psychology just don't apply to us. We've all heard things like "Ninety-nine percent of the time the thing you're worrying about won't happen" or "Think about all the good things that could happen instead of worrying." But once you've seen all the bad things that happen, you can never unsee them. If "ignorance is bliss," as the saying goes, does that mean awareness is anxiety? Parents of disabled children have had the veil of naivete lifted, and we're acutely aware of suffering and struggle. But does that mean it's hopeless? Does that mean that we're doomed to a life of anxious misery? Absolutely not. I've found that so much of managing my anxiety is in really understanding it, almost befriending it, and knowing when and how it's going to get triggered. Anxiety is our body's reaction to stress, and parenting is stressful. But we cannot (note: we SHOULD not) exist in a state of prolonged chronic stress.

The Function of Anxiety

To really understand how to battle anxiety, we must understand its function and role in our lives. Walk back in time with me to the Paleolithic era. You've got your cozy cave (this was long before Restoration Hardware, so you're roughing it), with a fire burning outside for warmth. You're gathered around the cave with your children while your partner is out hunting. Suddenly, you notice something move in the brush. You look closely and make out intricate black and yellow spots, and you quickly realize it's a hundred-pound leopard, and he's hungry. Very quickly, your cardiovascular system kicks into overdrive. Your blood pressure increases to pump blood to your heart and your concentration zones in on the animal. Your body is working to put you in prime condition to protect yourself and your family from the deadly leopard.

You instinctively position yourself in front of your children and raise your arms up over your head to intimidate the animal. You walk toward him and clap your hands to try to scare him away, and amazingly, it works! Your body did exactly what it needed to do to keep you and your children safe. Your fellow community members (cave cul-de-sac?) celebrate with a huge feast and party the night away in gratitude.

This stress response is actually meant to serve you by kicking your body into gear. When the perceived threat involves your child being sick (at its core, your brain is thinking all about death in those moments) rather than a leopard about to pounce, you have to consider how to care for your child and then how to calm your anxiety.

Coming up with a care plan for emergencies is a helpful way to take appropriate action when your child is sick. For example, if your child is prone to seizures, it's helpful to have a clear, written plan that's been co-created with your child's neurologist. I recommend that you have it typed out, in a binder, with clear step-by-step instructions on what medication to administer, when/if you should call for emergency help, and what to do once the seizure has stopped. Your anxiety wants to take action. This clear plan gives you something to do.

But what about when there is no emergency? What about when your child is at school and you can't stop ruminating about something bad happening? Many of us struggle with intrusive thoughts. An intrusive thought is an unwanted and uncontrollable image or thought that causes you distress. You're especially vulnerable to intrusive thoughts if you have a history of trauma. You might be sitting at work and suddenly become overwhelmed at the thought of your child having a medical emergency at school. These are often the moments that feel hardest to manage because your body has perceived a threat but there is really nothing you can do. There is no leopard to fight or fire to put out.

Battling Anxious Thoughts

You don't have to be at the mercy of your anxiety. You can use evidence to challenge an intrusive thought. What proof is there to support your thought? What proof is there to disprove it? For example, if you're worried your child might be sick at school, consider how your child was behaving that morning. Did they have a fever? Did it seem like they might be coming down with an illness? Acknowledge that your anxious mind is naturally skeptical, so you may have to seek a second opinion to get the full picture of reality. Maybe it's helpful to ask your partner how your child was acting before school. Fact-check, and then fact-check again. If after fact-checking you determine there's not much evidence to support your anxiety, remind yourself there's no threat and that it's okay to feel safe and let your guard down. If the answer is yes, move on to taking action.

If there is evidence to support your intrusive thought, consider what action you can take. Using the example from above, you could check in with the school to see how your child is doing. It's okay to email the teacher (within reason, of course). Most teachers of disabled children are used to frequent parental communication because of this exact reason. The caveat is that seeking reassurance must be practiced in moderation. If you find yourself needing to email your child's teacher every day to check in, you probably need to find a more sustainable solution. I again want to acknowledge here that this is especially difficult because many disabled children are chronically ill. It's sometimes legitimately difficult to identify when your child is sick. But part of the work of battling your anxiety is coexisting with your emotions and being able to self-soothe.

Once you have received reassurance, accept it. If the teacher emails you back and says your child is doing great, believe them. If your anxiety kicks up again, remind yourself of the evidence. The teacher responded and said all is well. Trust that the teacher would reach out to you if your child seemed off. It's a mental battle, but you can't let anxiety take the driver's seat.

Practice radical acceptance. Remember this concept from chapter 2? When you practice radical acceptance, you are making a conscious decision to accept the parts of your life that are not in your control (such as the uncertainty about your child's health). Radical acceptance involves confronting reality, regardless of your feelings about it. It's not about looking for a silver lining or forcing a smile when you're not feeling happy. You may dislike the situation, such as the anxious thoughts swirling in your mind, but instead of resisting them, you simply acknowledge them as they are. It's about allowing the waves of discomfort to wash over you without being overwhelmed, and allowing yourself to be present with your pain.

Focus on a mantra. A few of my favorites are "I've gotten through this before," "I trust the people who are taking care of my child," and "I am safe at this moment." Find the phrase that speaks to you, and say it over and over while loosening your shoulders and relaxing your muscles.

You can try mindfulness techniques that can bring your mind back to the present moment: deep breathing, focusing on three things you can see in the room, or holding an ice cube in your hand and focusing on the sensation. Anxiety experts often suggest exercise and spending time in nature as well. I've had success with both of these but am usually not able to engage in either when I'm knee-deep in an anxious moment. The key is to find what works for you. If a spin class helps ground you and release some anxiety, go for it. Take an active role in learning how you can soothe your anxiety and do something to make yourself feel better.

How to Self-Soothe During Anxious Times

You've likely heard the term *self-soothe*, which may sound easy but can actually be quite difficult, especially when your body is rarin' to go for some prime-time anxiety. Imagine you have a baby and she's crying. What would you do to soothe her? Probably pick her up, bounce her a bit, maybe make a calming "shhhhhh" noise. All of these are tried-and-true methods of soothing a baby. But what works for an adult—say, a forty-year-old woman in the throes of a panic attack fueled by health anxiety?

This is where self-awareness comes into play. My favorite question to ask clients is "What brings you joy?" You'd be surprised by how many people really struggle to answer that question. Your answer to this question can offer some insight into how you self-soothe. For me, a long walk outside with my dog and a great podcast is like balm to my soul. A deep chat with a friend, live music, and snuggling with my kids, husband, or dog—these are the things that soothe my nervous system.

So, I'll ask you this: When do you feel safe? When is your body at ease? What part of your answer can you intentionally implement in your daily life, especially when you notice yourself feeling anxious?

If you feel most relaxed at the beach yet you live in Nevada, can you get a gorgeous painting of the beach and fall asleep to the sound of waves every night? You have to work with what you have, obviously, but I encourage you to get creative and explore what brings you joy.

Anticipating Your Anxiety

For a long time, I felt beholden to my anxiety. I really believed it would be impossible to experience a medical emergency without falling apart. Anytime Asher showed even the slightest sign of sickness, I wouldn't be able to eat or function until I was sure he was completely healthy again. I am far from healed and still believe that we never fully "get over" health anxiety, but I have learned how to take some meaningful steps toward progress.

Take for example, Asher's recent spinal fusion surgery. He hasn't had many inpatient stays, but I knew this one would be an intense surgery and recovery. It ended up being a six-hour surgery and Asher was in the hospital for four nights. Obviously, not all hospital stays are anticipated, but since this one was, I was able to plan what I'd need to manage my anxiety and thus be able to be present for Asher.

To begin with, I wanted to plan who would spend the nights at the hospital. I was willing to do the overnights but felt anxious about the first couple of nights after surgery because it felt like there was a higher likelihood for a complication to arise during that time. After talking this over with my husband, we agreed that he would spend the first couple of nights with Asher, and if he needed a break, I'd take over after that. I planned to be at the hospital all day and give my husband a break to go home, and I also had a couple of friends who agreed to sit with me if I needed any extra support.

Did I feel guilty for not sleeping at the hospital? Yes (big yes!). A judgmental part of my brain told me that I was abandoning my child or that the nurses were probably judging me because I wasn't there 24/7.

But a more compassionate part of me reminded me that I deserved self-care and tenderness too. Asher was the one going through a major surgery, but I was witnessing my child going through a major surgery, and being partly responsible for taking care of him too. My back didn't feel pain, but my body was exhausted and my heart was weary from watching my child suffer. I vowed to take care of myself so that I could show up for him as the best version of me.

Making this simple plan and knowing that I had support and wouldn't have to spend the first couple of nights at the hospital eased a lot of my anxiety going into the surgery. We're not able to approach every situation this way, but when we can anticipate our anxiety, it helps us identify how to practice self-care in ways that are much more meaningful than a pedicure or glass of wine. I'm talking about real, restorative, reparative self-care that allows us to keep showing up for our kids without burning out.

Pursuing Therapy

I hate therapy.

Let me clarify. I love therapy when I'm the therapist, but I hate it when I'm the client. Just to begin, it takes so much effort to find a therapist who has openings that works with your schedule, and if you're hoping for someone in-network with your insurance, good luck! Therapy is often uncomfortable and hard, especially for someone like me who has a difficult time being vulnerable. But the times when I have committed to therapy consistently have been reparative and insightful. And as a therapist, I have witnessed so many clients mend their broken hearts in therapy. Therapy isn't a magic wand; it doesn't just fix things, but it can slowly shift your perspective or empower you to take action in areas that might need to be changed.

I often hear people say things like "I don't need therapy, I just talk to my friends," and while that may work in some cases, your friends aren't trained in the same ways as a therapist. A therapist is trained to look for patterns in behavior and thinking and offer insight in ways that move you toward your goals. Unlike a therapist, a friend is not a neutral person. They may have their own thoughts and opinions that are influenced by your relationship or their perspective on your situation. In therapy, you and your therapist will co-create goals, such as reducing anxiety in specific situations, improving communication skills with family members, setting boundaries with loved ones, or processing trauma from the birth or sickness of your child.

I found therapy to be especially helpful when I was pregnant with my second son and my anxiety was at an all-time high. This was also right around the time when I started taking medication for my anxiety. For me, an SSRI (selective serotonin reuptake inhibitor) has been helpful. A therapist can help you determine if medication is right for you and make a referral to a psychiatrist for a prescription if needed. You also can discuss medication with your general practitioner.

Finding a therapist who gets your situation can be a huge hurdle to obtaining meaningful therapy. While I'm confident that most graduate schools set up new therapists to be competent and prepared for most clients, parenting a disabled child is such a life-changing experience that it's sometimes hard to feel understood in therapy. I certainly don't believe that a therapist needs to have gone through the

Finding a Therapist You Trust:
What the Research Says

Study after study underscores the significance of a positive therapeutic relationship (the bond between client and therapist) in generating positive therapy outcomes. In fact, the alliance between client and therapist surpasses the significance of the type of therapy. This highlights the importance of finding a therapist with whom you feel a strong sense of trust. The therapist should not be a friend but rather a trusted figure who can gently challenge you, offer insight, and provide a safe space for your growth.

same experiences as their clients in order to fully understand them, but the all-consuming nature of parenting a disabled child is especially complicated. I personally found therapy difficult at times because the therapist often didn't fully grasp my son's disability, even though I'd tried to explain it over and over. Having a disabled child impacts every part of my life, from finding a babysitter to my ability to focus at work. Anytime the therapist would casually suggest a date night or some time away, I just felt more and more unseen—if only it were that easy!

My clients inspire me every day, but I remember one client in particular who was struggling with infertility. In her intake email she asked, "I hate to be so forward, but are you pregnant? Because that's not really something I can handle in a therapist at the moment."

This email has stuck with me because I loved how direct she was. It reminded me that it's okay to be direct about what you need and what you don't need in a therapist. Advocate for yourself the same way you do for your child. You're worth it!

Questions to Ask a Potential Therapist

- Have you worked with parents of disabled children before?

- Have you worked with disabled people before?

- What are your thoughts on disability? (This will tell you a lot about the therapist's knowledge, understanding, and unconscious biases about disability, all of which will greatly impact your work together.)

- Do you think it's appropriate for a person to feel grief in parenting a disabled child?

- What's your cancellation policy for emergencies?

- Can we switch to virtual sessions if we need to occasionally?

- Are you in-network with my insurance?

Over the years, I've come to better understand anxiety as my life-long companion. To be honest, I can't imagine a life without it, because despite all the work I've done, anxiety has never fully gone away. I used to be overcome with dread anytime anxiety settled in, but now I'm able to meet it with compassion and curiosity. Instead of being afraid, I consider what my anxiety needs in order to be soothed. There are still times when I can't eat, have digestive issues, or just fall into a puddle of tears because the anxiety is too overwhelming, but those times are few and far between. I'm a work in progress and parenting has left a permanent mark on me, and my guess is the same can be said for you. Maybe when it's all said and done, the most self-compassionate way to live with anxiety is simply to acknowledge what it's trying to tell us and then in turn understand how we can use that information as a barometer for true self-care.

Reflection Activity

Creating an Emergency Self-Care Plan

Imagine a time in the future when your child might experience something that will heighten your anxiety. Imagine something that, on a scale of 1 to 10, pushes your anxiety to an 8 or higher. Now, consider what you'll feel. Perhaps your emotions will include panic, fear, dread, anxiety, and isolation; write down anything that comes to mind.

Once you've labeled your potential emotions, brainstorm what might help comfort or regulate you. For example, if you're at the hospital, would it be helpful to have a friend sit with you or for you and your partner or other family member to take turns being at the hospital? Will you need breaks where you're able to go home and sleep, shower, work out, or just be outside and see the sunshine? Or will you feel better if you're at the hospital the entire time? If that's the case, what kind of food (besides hospital food) would you prefer? Could you call a friend and ask them to drop off some groceries or your favorite take-out meal?

Think about your support system and identify which people you could ask to help you in this scenario. If it helps, check in with your support system and ask people if you can put them on your short list of supporters for this sort of emergency.

Congratulations! You've started your emergency care plan. Now, when you notice yourself getting anxious about the possibility of this situation arising, remind yourself that you have a plan and you have support. You won't have to navigate this situation alone.

CHAPTER 8

Caring for Your Marriage

Most couples aren't emotionally, financially, or mentally prepared for the responsibility of parenting a disabled child. Your everyday premarital couple's session does not include scenarios about arguing with your health insurance company or finding the right pediatric surgeon or who's going to change the G-tube next. Couples enter marriage with hopes about how their life will look: white picket fence, 2.5 kids, and a dog (or some variation of the fairy tale). Rarely does that dream involve choosing medical devices for their child or making major medical decisions for an adult dependent. When hopes and expectations for parenthood are replaced with the uncertainty of parenting a disabled child, partners can struggle to cope. Our parenting journey fundamentally changes us, and those changes influence how we connect to and communicate with our partners.

As both a therapist and the mother to a disabled child, I quickly realized that parents needed help from someone who really understood the unique complexities of parenting. Very quickly, intake emails from couples needing help adjusting to parenting a disabled child overwhelmed my inbox. Over the years, I've had the privilege of working with many couples in the trenches of grief and anxiety while simultaneously trying to balance some sort of functional relationship. Each new couple on my couch gave me a deeper understanding of the complex connection between ourselves as individuals and our roles and struggles in marriage.

In this chapter, you'll meet three couples at different points in their parenting journey. Each partner has their own unique way of coping with their emotions, and those patterns are often rooted in their previous life experience and family of origin. You'll relate to some and possibly feel irritated by others. But like everyone, each person is struggling with adapting to their unmet expectations and fears around what it means to be a parent to a child with a disability.

Avoiding Hard Emotions: Alyssa and James

Most of us enter marriage with varying levels of comfort when it comes to expressing emotions. Our family of origin and early experiences often shape our narratives around what feelings are safe to express. The old adage is often true: Opposites do attract, which means your partner may avoid expressing the very emotions you feel most comfortable with. Many people are raised to believe that certain emotions (sadness, fear, vulnerability, to name a few) are an indicator of weakness and will go to lengths to protect themselves. As we know, the experience of parenting a child with a disability is one that stirs up many emotions, which can be a source of conflict for many couples as they try to work through their experiences in a connective way.

• • •

It was a typical Thursday, my busiest day in the office. I had a new couple at 2:00 p.m., and their intake paperwork mentioned that they had a child with what they labeled as "severe autism." I picked at my turkey sandwich and then used the restroom, returning to my office with just two minutes to spare. Almost immediately I heard the familiar buzz, alerting me that my clients had arrived.

Alyssa and James sat in front of me on the pale pink couch. We began our session with introductions, going over confidentiality and expectations. Very quickly, the topic of their daughter came up.

"It's been a hard road. Grace is four, and the baby is ten months. Grace is nonverbal. I mean, she communicates with us, but it's hard to know what she's thinking," Alyssa began.

"She's considered level 3," James added.

I nodded, understanding what this meant. Autism is categorized into three levels of function, with 1 needing the least support and 3 needing the most.

"But she's doing well," James continued. "It's hard at times, but we love her so much, and I know she's capable of anything."

"I've taken a leave of absence from work since we got her diagnosis. It's been seven months since I've worked," Alyssa said. "It's just too much—organizing her care and driving her to the therapy center after preschool each day. There's no way I can work. We're considering having my younger sister move in with us. We just need extra hands around here."

Alyssa reached for a tissue and dabbed at the corner of her eyes. James reached over and rested his hand on her leg. "Hey, it's okay. It's going to be okay," he reassured her. I could sense his anxiety rise as Alyssa expressed emotion, and Alyssa was clearly not reassured by James's response.

"And this is where we are," Alyssa said, shaking her head. "He always tells me it's going to be okay. But it's not. It's not okay."

James removed his hand from her leg and shook his head. "What am I supposed to say? She is so doom-and-gloom about it all. Do I wish our child didn't have autism? Yes. But what can we do about it? We have to stay positive."

I stopped them. "Can both exist at the same time? Why do you have to be doom-and-gloom or positive? Is it possible we can acknowledge the good and the bad together?"

It was clear that James was holding hope for the couple. He was acting as the cheerleader. But as I often see with couples, when one partner is holding so tight to one emotion, the other partner defaults to the exact opposite. I knew I needed Alyssa to acknowledge some hope and James to own his grief for this couple to break out of their cycle.

The process would take time. There are many reasons why it's hard to see the gray area in parenting. For those who default to positivity, that feeling sometimes protects against the reality of the situation. There's this misconception that if we allow space for complex emotions, we give up on our child. I knew that was what James was experiencing. He wanted to be a cheerleader for his child, which is not

How Did Your Family of Origin Handle Emotions?

Take this brief assessment to determine what messages about emotions might have been modeled for you in your family of origin. Once you answer the questions, reread your answers and see if you can pull out any common themes. Does your ability to express emotion mimic that of your parents, or have you developed new patterns?

These questions ask about your parents (plural), but consider them for each parent individually, or for whoever was your primary caretaker as you were growing up.

1. Can you remember a time when your parents were sad? How did they show they were sad?

2. When your parents were angry, how did they treat the rest of the family?

3. How did your parents respond when you were sad or hurt?

4. Did your parents interact with boy children differently from girl children? If so, how?

5. Did your family talk about emotions? Did you feel safe expressing your emotions in your family?

6. Now that you're an adult, do you find certain emotions safer than others to express?

bad—but it doesn't always allow much room for grief. And often, based on how emotion is expressed in our family of origin and other factors, we might think that sadness and anger are bad feelings.

There's a general cultural stigma (remember, good vibes only!) around admitting when we're feeling complex emotions, but the stigma around certain emotions begins long before parenthood. Early experiences in our family of origin often lay the foundation for how we understand and express emotion, and in particular whether we label specific emotions as bad, which is why I often ask clients how complex emotions were expressed in their families. The answer offers insight into someone's comfort level with openly expressing emotion.

After a few sessions with Alyssa and James, I explored this concept. James began to unpack how his family of origin may have contributed to his difficulty expressing certain emotions.

"James, can you tell me about a time when you felt sad? How did your family react?" I asked.

He thought for a moment. Then he said, "My grandfather died when I was young, probably about three. I don't remember meeting him, but there are a few pictures of us together. My mom always said that he was just sick; no other explanation was given. For some reason, I never really questioned that."

James went on to explain that he was assigned a family tree project in high school and had to get more information about exactly how his grandfather died.

"My mom was instantly so weird about it," he began. "I couldn't put it together, but I knew he wasn't just sick. Eventually, in a very roundabout way, she told me that he had killed himself and that he had been depressed for much of her childhood."

James said that his grandfather was always described as outgoing and happy and that deep down inside, his mother felt immense guilt about how he died. She found it too painful to talk about his grandfather's suicide, so the family generally avoided the topic. The subtle messaging was clear: Don't bring up grief because these feelings are too much to handle.

As we continued to talk, I asked James how this family rule about not bringing up certain emotions impacts him as Grace's dad. I wanted to know if it affected his ability to express his emotions related to parenting a disabled child.

"I don't know," he said, and then stopped to think for a moment. "I guess I still kind of believe that if I show sadness, I'm doing something bad. I don't want Alyssa to be weighed down by my sadness. Even more than that, I never want Grace to see me sad about her disability. I want her to know that I believe in her and love her exactly how she is."

"And if you're sad about her disability, that will show her otherwise?" I asked.

"It feels like it would," he said.

Maybe James couldn't change his instinct to dismiss any feelings of sadness around his daughter's diagnosis. Still, he was beginning to see how he masked his grief as denial and positivity. He was slowly unraveling the subtle ways in which vulnerable emotions were discouraged when he was growing up and how that impacted his experience of parenting as an adult.

Measuring the Effect on Marriages

There have been conflicting data over the years, but you've probably heard that parents of disabled children have a higher divorce rate than parents of nondisabled children. However, data pulled from the Wisconsin Longitudinal Study, which spanned 50 years and followed 190 couples who had a disabled child, proved this age-old myth wrong. The study found no increased risk of divorce in couples with disabled children. One interesting finding was that in families with nondisabled children, the risk of divorce increased as the number of children increased; however, in families with a disabled child, the fewer children in the family, the higher the likelihood of divorce. In other words, in families with a disabled child, additional siblings served as a protective factor for the marriage.

Past experiences with and conditioning around emotions set the foundation for how partners express themselves in relationships. Learning that a child has an unexpected diagnosis brings up powerful feelings, and parents often have to unlearn the subtle messaging they received as children about how and when to express them. Learning to accept feelings without judgment can feel unnatural, but it can also lead to self-acceptance and, ultimately, a deeper connection with others, including our spouse or partner.

The Separation of Church and State: Jerome and Tasha

While some people cope with the stress of parenting a disabled child by using positive thinking to avoid emotions, others are quite the opposite. Some people want to dive into their parental role and spend every spare moment learning about available treatments for their disabled child and connecting to other parents with similar situations. We can call this type "the researcher." This person is motivated by the desire to help their child thrive and to learn as much as possible, but that desire can quickly consume their entire identity, leaving little room for a healthy marriage. The other partner in this situation usually feels incompetent and leans into work or other interests to find their identity.

This dynamic is exactly why I encourage couples to try to find times when they can practice separation of church and state—that is, church being the marriage, and state being the responsibilities that come from parenting a disabled child. Healthy couples need occasional breaks from problem-solving and advocating, as well as times when they can connect emotionally and sexually and feel united as both partners and parents.

• • •

Jerome and Tasha found themselves in couples therapy as they approached their nineteenth wedding anniversary. Their son Pierce had cerebral palsy. He used a wheelchair independently but needed assistance with bathing, feeding, and communicating. Pierce had just turned thirteen, and Jerome and Tasha were beginning to research high schools for their son. I quickly discovered that Tasha was the researcher in the relationship.

"Tell me, where are you in the high school application process?" I asked.

Tasha started, saying, "We're going to tour specialized and traditional schools. But we can't decide what's best for Pierce. I've read a million different opinions and can't seem to decide. It'd be nice if I had some support and wasn't the only one trying to figure it out."

"Oh, come on," responded Jerome. "I've tried. I don't have hours to spend at the computer. I'm not even on social media, and you're asking all your friends in your groups for opinions. Whenever I try to offer my opinion, you disagree with me. As you know, I'd prefer to send him to a specialized school where we know he's safe and the teachers know how to work with him."

"Yeah, well, I like the idea of him being around nondisabled friends and being in a more integrated setting. And for the record, I don't spend hours researching every night," Tasha said.

"Really? You don't? I went to bed at eleven o'clock last night, and when I woke up a couple of hours later, you were still out in the living room on your laptop." Jerome then explained that he had wanted Tasha to come to bed earlier but knew she was in the research zone. He eventually acknowledged his gratitude for all she did but said that he often felt neglected and out of the loop.

As our sessions went on, it became clear that Tasha felt immense pressure to manage everything related to her son. Jerome felt forgotten and incapable of caring for Pierce in a way that would please Tasha. Jerome expressed sadness about the changes in their relationship, including a nonexistent sex life for the past two years.

I felt a massive amount of compassion for Tasha. Her mental load was overwhelming. Pierce required constant care, and most of that responsibility fell on her. But I couldn't blame Jerome for how he felt. He missed Tasha. Over time, Tasha had put all her energy into parenting and had lost touch with her marriage. Of course, Tasha and Jerome were equally responsible for the drift that had occurred over the years. Both partners assumed their respective roles, each necessary to keep the family afloat. There just wasn't a lot of extra energy to give to their relationship.

While the divorce rates in parents of disabled children aren't necessarily higher than in parents of nondisabled children, it's easy to see

Creative Dating When Childcare Is Hard to Find

For the parent of a disabled child, a good babysitter is worth their weight in gold—and the price you'll pay for a night out reflects that value. It's no secret that many disabled kids have unique needs, and not just anyone can meet those needs. A disabled child may have a feeding tube, wheelchair, or other assistive devices and specific communication needs or require medical assistance throughout the day. The challenges faced in finding trustworthy childcare are unique and often misunderstood, but they are very real.

Couples may need to harness creativity to find time for connection. Perhaps date night used to entail reservations at a new restaurant, but now it's pizza and wine at home after your child goes to bed. A date might mean meeting midday while school is in session (take advantage of that consistent childcare!). You might take a walk together in the park while your child is in speech therapy. You might even have sex in the middle of the night just because it's the only time that works (I know those of you with kids who don't sleep well are shaking your head in anger reading this!). What's most important is that couples find a way to prioritize time with each other. This is not just a luxury but a necessity for maintaining a healthy relationship. By making their connection with each other a priority, parents can ensure that they are on the path to a strong and enduring bond.

how couples can drift apart and start to lead separate lives. The struggle is real for all parents, but parents of disabled children tend to have a heavier load and the added stress of constantly advocating for their child.

I wanted to better understand what connected Tasha and Jerome before their world revolved around caring for their son. In a later session I asked them to reflect on life before they became parents.

"We used to have a lot of fun," Tasha said as she looked at Jerome and raised her eyebrows. We all laughed. The energy in the room softened.

"Remember when we got kicked out of the movie theater? We were supposed to be watching *Harry Potter* but really we were making out." Jerome put his arm around Tasha, and she leaned into him. For a brief moment, I saw the spark. I saw a version of Tasha and Jerome that made me feel like going home and passionately kissing my husband. I, too, remembered those days before parenting consumed us.

"I want you to go out on a date and try your best to not talk about Pierce," I said. "I'm not saying you have to go make out in a movie theater, but try to get back in touch with the things that made you fall in love twenty-some years ago."

"I love the idea, but it seems almost impossible," Tasha said. "But I want to try it. We'll plan in advance and see if we can find a sitter."

• • •

A few weeks later, in a follow-up session, I wanted to know more about Tasha's assumed role as the researcher in the relationship.

"Tasha, can you tell me how it feels to be the one doing most of the researching and caretaking for Pierce?" I asked.

Tasha paused before speaking. "As soon as he was born, I was on Google. I read all about therapies before he was even home from the NICU. I joined a Facebook group with other parents of kids with CP. I wanted to talk about it with Jerome all the time. I felt like the more I researched, the better mom I'd be. It felt like something I could actually do when everything else was out of my control."

Jerome explained that he found meaning through his work and often stayed late at the office. Tasha was so competent in managing Pierce's needs that Jerome felt useless when it came to parenting. But this dynamic took a toll on both partners.

"If caring for Pierce is my thing, I'm forced to do it alone. That pisses me off. It shouldn't be my thing. I feel so burned out. The burden is so overwhelming. I feel like I'm going to miss something," Tasha said.

I asked Tasha what she needed from Jerome to feel like they were equal partners in parenting.

"I need it to become his thing too. I need him to go to doctor's appointments. I need him to have the important phone numbers in his phone. I need him to email teachers and reorder medications. Should I go on?" Tasha smiled.

Jerome expressed that he was willing to jump in and share the load but needed Tasha to loop him in. They agreed to create a shared calendar and to-do list so that they could be more in sync about what was going on with Pierce and with each other.

Over time, we worked on the division of labor and mental load in Tasha and Jerome's relationship. It took work. Tasha had difficulty trusting that Jerome would hold up his end of the deal. She was so used to micromanaging everything that it was hard to let go. She had to find flexibility in her expectations. Tasha would schedule an appointment the second she thought of it, but Jerome needed to write a sticky note and call the next day. Either way, it got done, and that was the important part. Jerome needed to focus on being engaged and making time in his schedule. This required him to talk to his boss and be more transparent about what was happening. He occasionally had to take time off work to go to appointments. It wasn't easy, but this new family structure positively impacted everything. Tasha's trust in Jerome increased. By more equally sharing the responsibility, Jerome felt more involved in parenting.

I encouraged Jerome and Tasha to practice intentional weekly check-ins. It sounds like such a simple concept, but amid life's chaos, many couples struggle to find time to connect. I encourage couples to find a consistent time each week to put the phones away, eliminate other distractions, and sit down to thoughtfully talk to each other and reflect on anything that might cause stress in the week ahead. This is also a great time to exchange information about schedules, updates, or important appointments. The partner least involved in researching or scheduling can actively ask questions and catch up so they aren't out of the loop. I encourage clients to go into these weekly check-ins with compassion and curiosity, focusing on how they can connect to their partner and help them feel supported.

The Urge to Numb Out: Tessa and Alexis

Sometimes the emotional and physical demands of parenting a disabled child are so overwhelming that parents feel the need to escape. Escaping can manifest in many ways: food, alcohol, drugs, physical or emotional affairs, working out, sleeping. Basically, anything that can provide respite from reality can be used to numb emotional pain. Perhaps home is chaotic due to a child's behavior or medical needs, so a parent works late hours to avoid the stress. Or perhaps a parent has an emotional affair with a coworker or old fling because it helps them feel happiness and desire. These behaviors usually come from a place of pain but can cause enormous damage and betrayal of trust in a relationship.

Numbing is a sign that you are disconnected from your body. Reconnecting with your body allows you to experience the full range of your emotions. For this reason, it's crucial to gradually incorporate mind-body activities into your routine. This could involve daily body scans, using a meditation app, journaling about your emotions, or seeking support from a therapist. Be kind to yourself, and remember, you've likely spent years avoiding the very feelings you're trying to confront. It will be tough, but what's even more challenging? Continuously avoiding your feelings!

How to Do a Body Scan

1. Find a comfortable spot and begin to notice your breathing. Notice the way the air fills your lungs and start to connect to how your body is feeling.

2. You can start with any body part, but I find it helpful to begin with my head. Notice how your head is feeling. Pay attention to the sensations on your scalp, on your face, near your ears, and around your jaw. Are you holding any tension in your head and face? Are you able to relax your muscles? Is anything hurting?

3. Move on to the next body part. I like to move on to my neck, chest, and stomach and then downward until I reach my feet. Do what feels best for you. Take inventory and notice the sensations, pain, muscle tension, and general well-being of your body parts.

4. If your mind wanders at any point (which is a normal part of the process!), bring your attention back to your breathing as an anchor to ground you.

• • •

Tessa and Alexis had always dreamed of adopting. They were thrilled when they matched with a birth mom and became moms to the baby of their dreams, Hazel. But when Hazel was four months old, she was diagnosed with Werdnig-Hoffmann disease, also known as spinal muscular atrophy (SMA) type 1. This complex syndrome can be terminal. Alexis and Tessa instantly pursued couples therapy.

The couple sat on the couch. Alexis rested her elbows on her knees and cupped one of Tessa's hands in both of hers. The room was quiet, with just the sound of my white noise machine humming steadily in the corner.

"I know this has been incredibly difficult. How are you both doing as you navigate this?" I asked.

Five Signs of Emotional Numbing

Emotional numbing, a common response to stress or trauma, is something many parents can relate to. In the whirlwind of our daily lives, it's not uncommon to find ourselves numbing our emotions to cope. Here are five signs that you might be doing so.

1. You feel a lack of emotion (pleasurable or unpleasant), regardless of how intense of a situation you're experiencing.

2. You experience constant fatigue, difficulty concentrating, and low motivation.

3. The activities or hobbies that used to bring you joy no longer matter to you.

4. You find it difficult to connect to the people you love.

5. You find yourself turning to harmful activities, such as drinking excessive amounts of alcohol, consuming drugs, or other addictions, like excessive gaming or binge-watching television shows.

Alexis began. "I don't even know what to say. We got the diagnosis three weeks ago. It's hard to explain how much our lives have been turned upside down. We waited years to find Hazel, and now it feels like we could lose her. Everything seemed so normal. The birth mom said she moved all the time, and everything looked normal in the ultrasounds. Everything seemed perfect." Tears began to stream down her face. She let go of Tessa's hand and buried her face in her hands. Tessa closed her eyes and cried as well. We sat in silence.

There's this misconception about therapists that we don't feel or express emotion in session. That we're a blank canvas. I fundamentally disagree with this outdated teaching. As a therapist, this was one of those moments where I couldn't contain my sadness. I felt hot tears roll down my face, brought back to that moment of Asher's diagnosis when my entire world changed. A phone call, a meeting with a geneticist, and my world was flipped upside down. Now I was sitting in front of two new parents who faced the same situation and were drowning in their own pain. They looked to me for some sense of guidance or hope.

"You're prioritizing your relationship in the middle of a hurricane. That shows such commitment to each other and to Hazel," I said.

"We're barely surviving," Tessa said. "I'm not sleeping or eating. I'm living off wine and the occasional bowl of cereal."

"And I'm worried about that. I'm worried about you. I'm worried about Hazel. Tessa is right. We're barely keeping it together," Alexis added.

I did my best to normalize what they were feeling. I wanted to hold space for both partners and their different coping methods. I quickly realized that Alexis was in action mode, scheduling doctor appointments, researching, and communicating with therapists. She'd found the closest hospital that could do the life-saving gene therapy that Hazel would soon begin. She was the partner who contacted me for a couple's therapy appointment. As the session went on, I noticed that Tessa was significantly depressed, and while that wasn't entirely abnormal, I didn't want it to go on for too long.

We met weekly, and in our fifth session, things started to take a turn for the worse. Our session was at 10:00 a.m., and Tessa and Alexis were usually prompt. At 10:10, I heard the buzzer and let the couple in. But Alexis walked in alone.

"Tessa isn't coming. She's hungover," Alexis stated.

"On a Tuesday at ten in the morning?" I asked, feeling instantly concerned.

"Yes. It's becoming more and more of a problem. It hasn't gotten in the way of her work until today. But she's drinking every night. I'm at a loss. I can't do this alone, and I'm so worried about Tessa. I also snuck a look at her phone and saw her sending Snapchats to her ex-girlfriend. I'm pissed and worried."

Alexis was overwhelmed. She was managing her own emotional reaction to Hazel's diagnosis, trying to create a structure for Hazel's care, and now pulling her partner out of a depression.

Earlier in this chapter, we met Tasha, whose identity was enmeshed with her role as the researcher. The opposite of that is the parent who cannot tolerate the demands of parenting and wants to escape entirely from it by numbing themselves. This behavior creates a complicated dynamic in a couple.

The numbing partner is often emotionally (and sometimes physically) absent or unable to step up as an equal partner. This means the entire load of parenting falls on their partner. The present partner becomes entrenched in caretaking, acutely aware of their child's every need and never getting a break, while the numbing partner goes on with their life, often spiraling out of control. This dynamic isolates partners from each other. It's important to note that this isn't a good guy/bad guy situation. The numbing partner usually doesn't have the coping skills to effectively face the emotional implications of parenting a disabled child; numbing is almost always an act of self-preservation. Before the numbing partner can engage in parenting, they must learn to manage their fears and emotions around parenting a disabled child.

I quickly connected Tessa to an individual therapist and both partners to an online support group for parents of babies with SMA. As our sessions continued, Tessa became more and more present in the relationship and parenting. She expressed that her biggest fear was losing Hazel and that it was just too much to face when she received the diagnosis. Tessa worked on acknowledging when she needed breaks and increasing her tolerance for uncertainty. She also attended sobriety support groups. She continued to struggle with the temptation to numb but was able to catch herself more times than not. We had a session shortly after Hazel had an inpatient stint at the hospital after battling a respiratory illness.

"This has been a tough stretch for you. What are you finding most helpful in navigating the uncertainty?" I asked.

Tessa replied, "My therapist has helped me learn the concept of radical acceptance. I've talked to Alexis ad nauseam about this, but I'm working toward simply accepting the diagnosis and recognizing that it's just part of Hazel's story. It doesn't mean I'm happy about SMA. I have a mantra on the hard days: 'I don't have to love it, but I do have to live with it.'"

Tessa's work was ongoing, but she was finding ways to be present as a partner and parent, and that was a big win.

We go into marriage as one version of ourselves, but the experience of parenting a disabled child can change us entirely. Where we once felt soft, we may now feel resentful and hard. Where we used to feel open and optimistic, we may now feel cynical and closed off. Then again, we may find new parts of ourselves that feel strong and capable. In a marriage, we must negotiate this new version of ourselves to fit with our partner's new version. Seeing and honoring our evolving selves and partners takes time and tenderness. But, at the end of the day, no one understands our unique experience as much as our partner and co-parent. Investing in our marriage is worth it and necessary.

Reflection Exercises

- Which parent do you relate to most in this chapter?

  - *Alyssa, who felt that her partner didn't allow her to feel certain emotions and needed to verbally process them*

  - *James, whose experience with his family of origin trained him to believe that certain emotions were off-limits and therefore was unable to freely express sadness about his child's diagnosis*

  - *Tasha, the researcher whose identity had become learning all the things*

  - *Jerome, who immersed himself in work because he felt iced out by his partner and longed to be closer to her*

- *Alexis, who sprang into action but felt abandoned by her partner*

- *Tessa, who struggled with numbing as a form of escaping the realities of her situation*

Couples Connection Exercise

Sit down with your partner and take turns talking for two to five minutes (uninterrupted) about what you appreciate about each other. When do you feel most loved by your partner? What is your partner good at? In a separate exercise (on a different day), take two minutes each and discuss what you need most from your partner. Be sure to use non-attacking words.

Date Night

Plan ahead and schedule a date with your partner, and remember, it's okay to get creative with what you're doing! Try to be intentional about discussing topics that aren't related to parenting. After, reflect on how it felt to be together and connect in ways that didn't revolve around your child.

CHAPTER 9

Growing Your Family

Johanna and her twelve-year-old daughter Sylvia scheduled a session with me because Sylvia had become growingly irritable at home. They wanted to work with me, specifically, because Sylvia had an older sister with a rare genetic syndrome. Sylvia was a happy and healthy kid. She got good grades at school, loved soccer and *Calvin and Hobbes*, and was overall well-adjusted. As we started talking about how having a disabled sister impacted her, Sylvia began to open up about her emotions.

"I just wish my sister didn't have a disability. I feel like I can never invite friends over to my house because it's embarrassing. She yells all the time, and the attention is always on her. I wish my sister had never been born," she confessed.

A look of hurt washed over Johanna's face as she shifted uncomfortably in her chair. "That's not a very nice thing to say," she said, looking down at her wringing hands.

I was about to intervene when Sylvia responded, "Mom. You told me to be honest. You can't get mad at me for saying that when you told me to be honest."

I knew that this moment was important. Johanna needed to be open to Sylvia's perspective. Sylvia's entire life had been shaped by having a sister with a disability. It impacted the attention she got from her parents, her ability to do extracurricular activities, her responsibilities at home, and so much more.

I paused for a moment to let Sylvia's words sink in. I simultaneously felt the urge to scold her and hug her. It was painful to hear her unfiltered feelings about some of the harder parts of having a disabled sibling, but at the same time, I understood what she was trying to convey. Having a disabled sibling affected so much of Sylvia's life, and she was allowed to have a reaction to it, especially in a safe space such as therapy. I was used to working with people with disabled family members, but rarely did someone come out and say something so brutal.

It took Johanna some time to let her guard down and hear Sylvia's words in a nondefensive way, but over time she was able to make some meaningful changes at home that helped Sylvia feel like she was allowed to take up more space. Johanna and her husband made a point to take Sylvia alone on outings where she could have their full attention. Johanna also started to become more aware of the ways in which she depended on Sylvia to be more grown up than she was and the amount of responsibility she put on her to (in her words) "keep an eye on" her sister. It wasn't that Sylvia resented this, but it subtly sent the message that she needed to be more responsible than most kids her age. Once Johanna made a point not to rely on Sylvia so heavily, it motivated Sylvia to offer to help more, because she felt like it wasn't expected of her.

Of course, not every nondisabled sibling is able to articulate their feelings as directly as Sylvia. Likewise, not every parent is open to hearing feedback. As parents, we must attune to the way we balance responsibility and attention when we have children of varying abilities.

We have to honestly assess our capabilities to meet the needs of our children, acknowledging that it's sometimes really hard to get this right. We are, of course, human, and we oftentimes look to our nondisabled child to help support and care for our disabled child. When this is done thoughtfully, with care and love, it can be a beautiful opportunity for our nondisabled child to have a tender and life-changing relationship with their sibling. Fostering this bond also teaches our nondisabled child to accept differences, care for others, and be more attuned to the need for advocacy for the rights of disabled people. It's not all sympathy and tenderness, though. I'm the mom of three boys, and though Asher has contributed to our family in valuable ways that impact each of us, my kids all argue with and tease one another just like any other siblings.

It is true, however, that parenting a disabled child can take up a lot of a parent's bandwidth. If we're not mindful, we might not have much energy left for other family members. If our child is in and out of the hospital or has a lot of therapies, we may spend a lot of our energy caretaking. And when we sense that one of our children is doing well and seems to have a good handle on their life, it's easy for us to assume they don't need extra care. The child that has the most obvious needs is oftentimes the one who receives most of our attention. But is this doing a disservice to our seemingly independent, emotionally healthy child? How do we remain proactive (not reactive) in how we meet our nondisabled child's needs, even if they don't seem to need us in the same way our disabled child does? How can we stay mindful of our nondisabled child's needs and allow space for their honest emotions, complexities, and maybe even resentment?

The responsibility of caring for a disabled child can take up much of our time and energy, ultimately leaving less for everyone else. In a perfect world, our family (perhaps including grandparents, friends, and extended family) would rally and collectively offer support, but we all know the world is far from perfect. Also, we know that children can't always be given the responsibility to care for their disabled sibling, and we cannot expect them to be self-sufficient before they're ready.

When it comes to the decision to have more children, many parents of a disabled child live in fear of what would happen if they had another disabled child simply because there is not enough energy, time, money, or attention to adequately care for multiple disabled children. All parents, regardless of their children's disability status, must make thoughtful decisions about what's right for their family, but when a disabled child is in the family, the stakes can be heightened because the caretaking may last forever.

To Have or Not to Have? That Is the Question.

Just like everyone else, parents of disabled children have all sorts of motivations for the ways in which we grow or don't grow our families. For some, practicality rules out the desire to have more children. Maybe the parents are happy with the number of children they have, whether that's one or more. Maybe their disabled child's needs require all their resources. Some parents are devastated to learn that one or both partners are carriers for a genetic syndrome and decide not to risk transmitting that syndrome to another child. Some parents live with the reality that their child has a terminal diagnosis and refuse to gamble with bringing into the world another child who may have the same condition.

There's grief involved when our expectations and dreams of growing our family are out of reach or when it feels like the decision of how many kids to have has been made for us. Even if it's subconscious, many of us grew up with an ideal image of what our family might someday look like. No one expects their family construct to be limited by genetic factors or having a child who requires full-time care forever.

Some parents take the opposite approach and are intent on having more children, fueled by all sorts of factors. Some parents simply want a big family and have the means to pursue that dream. Parents might make the decision to adopt or foster a child, acknowledging that they want more children but that the risk involved in having another biological child is too much. Some parents even intentionally have more children so they can someday have help caring for their disabled child (a complex decision, to say the least).

The Four Fs of Family Planning

Lauren Rizzo, the mom of a disabled child, suggests that parents who are struggling with the decision to have more children take a serious look at what she calls "the Four Fs": finances, flexibility, fairness, and family. Exploring these factors in your life can help you determine if you have the bandwidth to have more children.

- **Finances** means whether or not you're able to afford another child given all the costs associated with parenting a disabled child. These could include medical bills, childcare, and necessary medical or assistive devices as well as the potential need for one partner to be a full-time caretaker rather than an income earner.

- **Flexibility** highlights the constant requirement to respond to your disabled child's needs. How flexible do you need to be? Is your child often hospitalized long-term? Would having another child make it impossible for you to adequately support your disabled child?

- **Fairness** focuses on your ability to parent *all* your children. Is it unfair to your disabled child for you to have more children? Would it be unfair to future children that so much of your energy goes toward your disabled child?

- **Family** represents outside support, or your village. Do you have adequate support for your potential future children if an emergency arises for your disabled child?

Examining these factors with your partner can help you make a wise decision related to growing your family in a responsible and compassionate way.

I want to be clear: None of this is easy. For many parents of a disabled child, the path to growing their family is complicated.

As we face the decision to have more children, we must take an honest look at our bandwidth and ability to adequately care for everyone involved. In the same way, once our families are complete, we must make a point to ensure that everyone feels seen, heard, and cared for. If we don't do this, we will cause harm to our children. The potential for parentifying our nondisabled children by giving them an inappropriate level of responsibility for their disabled sibling is high, and as parents, we have to be attuned to this dynamic.

Glass Child Syndrome

Consistently, parents I've spoken with often share that they want to have more children in part to be a support system for their disabled child. When a disabled child is reliant on their parent as their forever caretaker, a parent can't help but wonder, "Who will care for my child when I'm gone?"

Siblings are often deeply impacted by having a disabled brother or sister and the expectations (sometimes unspoken) that they themselves should not add to the stress of the family. But these expectations can place tremendous pressure on a nondisabled sibling, leading to resentment and, ultimately, glass child syndrome. A glass child is labeled as such because they receive the messaging, either directly or indirectly, that they aren't allowed to take up space or contribute to the chaos of the home—in essence, they come to feel that they are expected to be invisible or see-through. Glass children may perceive that their disabled or sick sibling takes up all of their parents' energy, and at the end of the day, there's no energy left for anyone else.

Jacob had never heard of the term *glass child*, but when I gave him the definition, he paused and said, "That was absolutely my life growing up."

Jacob was the middle child of three. His older sister was in and out of trouble and his younger brother, Parker, was profoundly disabled, born with agenesis of the corpus callosum. This impacted Parker's communication, mobility, and vision. Jacob's mom and dad divorced when he was in middle school, which left him spending his time primarily with his mom.

Jacob doesn't remember the first time his mom referred to him as her angel, but she did it often, and its effect on Jacob was complicated. "I was the easy one to raise, but my mom subtly sent the message that it needed to be that way. Between my brother's and my sister's needs, there wasn't much room for me to exist. My role was to be the angel. Don't add to the stress and do whatever I can to make my mom's life easier," Jacob said.

Anytime he did struggle, he felt like his mother didn't have the bandwidth to validate his feelings. "I'm not sure if it's because she had to maintain a positive mindset, but I've never perceived my mom as someone who processes her emotions very well. Her motto is always 'everything is going to be okay.' She couldn't acknowledge how hard things really were. This still persists to this day," he told me.

Jacob can still see the many ways in which his mom was a good parent. He's able to recognize that she was handling a massive number of demands on her energy and time as the single parent of three kids, two of whom were especially high-need. He also remembers that she was at every single one of his sporting events and was always willing and able to drive him to his many activities.

"My mom gave me a lot of attention in the way she was capable of, and I believe she did the best she could," he said. "In many ways she was a great mother. Physically she was always there. But emotionally—she just didn't have the tools to provide what I needed. Looking back, I can clearly see that she used my brother to be a distraction from emotions."

When I asked him what he wishes his parents would have done differently, Jacob didn't miss a beat: "I wish my parents were more emotionally present. I wish they would have given me space to feel. Every parent wants their kid to be happy, but the truth is it's normal to feel unhappy. I wish my parents were present for me and allowed me to have those feelings instead of always saying everything was going to

Validating Our Nondisabled Children's Feelings

Our children have a way of being attuned to what we are feeling, even if we're not verbally expressing emotions. Children know when we're distracted or annoyed and learn to respond to our nonverbal cues. It's important that we invite our nondisabled kids into conversations about how they're doing and what they need. If our child gives us feedback that is hard to hear (like when my client Sylvia told her mother that she wished her brother wasn't disabled), it's essential that we do not take a defensive stance in our response. If we shame our child for giving honest feedback, they will be less likely to do so in the future.

Validating emotions and inviting more conversation looks like:

- I know that having a disabled sibling can be hard at times. Let's talk about what I can do to help you feel more comfortable at home.

- I can see that you're feeling mad. Let's talk about it.

- How do you think having a disabled sibling affects you as a member of our family?

- Is there anything you wish I did differently when it comes to balancing your and your siblings' needs?

be okay. That's probably the biggest reason why I'm not close to my mom now—because she can't tolerate the spectrum of normal human emotions."

When I met with Jacob and heard about his experience, I was able to hold compassion for both him and his mother. As the parent of three kids, I'm always trying to practice the art of meeting everyone's needs, and I don't always get it right. Parents of multiple children with varying abilities must be aware of the pressure they put on their nondisabled children to minimize their needs. We do this in subtle ways, but we do it. It's easy to feel so overwhelmed with the demands of parenting a disabled child that, whether implicitly or explicitly, we ask our other children not to add to our load. If you're reading this and feeling a sense of guilt wash over you, notice it. Notice the feeling and take a moment to offer yourself some compassion. For many of us, our nondisabled children can navigate the world with more independence than our disabled children. But that doesn't mean they don't need us. Their ability to handle chaos and be flexible doesn't mean they won't mess up or get into trouble, just like any other child. We have to make space for our nondisabled children to be just that: children.

When it comes to having a disabled child in the family, remember that a parent's experience will be very different from a sibling's experience. Our children will likely experience their disabled sibling as (gasp!) just their sibling! As parents, we influence how our kids view one another, including a disabled sibling, and it's important to foster healthy relationships between all siblings, regardless of their abilities.

Doug Koonce was a year and a half old when his younger brother Jon was born. Jon was injured during birth and had cerebral palsy with high support needs. "Jon and I grew up as really good companions," Doug said. "He didn't use words, but I learned that communication doesn't always require words. I asked questions and he had a sound for yes and a sound for no."

Doug and Jon shared a bedroom for many years, but even after they got separate rooms, Doug found himself sleeping on Jon's floor just because he liked being close to him. As he recalled, "His personality was lighthearted. He'd always get my attention anytime certain commercials came on TV because we had inside jokes about them." Doug now realizes that his brother was aiming for connection through these sweet interactions.

"After Jon died," Doug said, "my mom apologized because I had to grow up in such a strange situation. She apologized for him. I hated that because having Jon as a brother didn't feel strange to me."

Upon reflection, Doug feels that his mom apologized for the wrong thing: "I was basically abandoned as a child. I would just go back in my room with the door locked and stay out of the way. I never wanted to make things worse, and I also had to take care of my mother because she had a lot going on. As an adult, I grapple with this mother wound."

Having Jon as a brother fundamentally shaped Doug's personality in many beautiful ways. Doug describes himself as empathic and attuned to people with any difference or disability. Doug deeply misses Jon and visits his grave at least once a month.

"Having Jon as my brother was just my normal. Jon was just Jon. I never ever saw him as a problem," Doug said.

What the Research Shows About Having a Disabled Sibling

One recent study suggests that growing up with a disabled sibling correlates with having higher levels of cognitive empathy. The study examined eleven-year-old twins, some with a nondisabled/disabled makeup, and others with a nondisabled/nondisabled makeup. The children who had a disabled sibling demonstrated higher levels of empathy than peers whose twin was not disabled.

Another study suggests that males with a disabled sibling are at a higher risk for experiencing emotional fragility. This study especially highlighted siblings of someone with autism or Down syndrome.

It's important to acknowledge that the data on having a sibling with a disability is not black-and-white, and many people with a disabled sibling express that their life felt stable and largely positive. The bottom line: Parents set the tone for whether their kids feel loved and included, regardless of ability status.

Congrats, You're Pregnant (and Anxious)!

For anyone who's had another child after having a disabled child, you know that the journey to holding that new baby in your arms is often filled with anxiety. I've never been more anxious than when I was pregnant with my second son, after Asher was born. Not only had my eyes been opened to what could go wrong, but I realized there were hundreds of worst-case scenarios. My baby had forty-six chromosomes, and any little piece that might be missing could cause a life-altering condition. In fact, I often told myself that we were lucky with Asher's diagnosis. His syndrome is compatible with life. Most people with Prader-Willi syndrome can be expected to live a full life, unlike so many other diagnoses. My anxiety soared as I considered every possible diagnosis or issue that could arise.

Despite my anxiety, everything with my second-born son felt easy. I got pregnant with Silas quickly, his birth was uneventful and healthy, and he even took his first steps a few weeks before he turned one. On paper you'd think this would have been the best time of my life, but it highlighted all that I'd missed out on with Asher. I suddenly realized what the early days of parenting were like for everyone else and how hard Asher had had to work for what seemed to come easily to every other baby. A deep grief for the experiences I'd never get to have with Asher, and for the difficulty and isolation of those early years with him, set in. I never had this perspective until I became a parent to a nondisabled child.

I will never take the ease of getting pregnant with Silas for granted. The rest of our story was not easy at all. My husband and I tried for years to get pregnant again, including a failed round of IVF. After IVF didn't work, I began to wonder if anyone with a disabled child had an easy road to having more children. Emotionally, mentally, genetically—somehow it all seems touched by the enormous weight of responsibility. But true to form, we learn to persist and fight tooth and nail for what we need. Family planning is no exception. Indeed, eventually we conceived and our third son, Jasper, joined our family.

Brittany Steitz walked away from her twenty-week ultrasound feeling more confused than reassured. Her unborn son had a spinal issue as well as a flattened nose, which could mean he had any number of abnormalities. Brittany eventually got an amniocentesis as well as an MRI, but before she could get the results of the amnio back, her biggest fear became a reality. Brittany's son Logan died in utero due to a brain bleed. She gave birth to him at twenty-six weeks of gestation and he had died three days before.

After the devastating loss of Logan, Brittany eventually learned that she was a carrier for a rare genetic syndrome. This was a shock to Brittany and her husband, as they already had an older child who was not impacted by the syndrome. Brittany and her husband wanted to have more children, but due to her carrier status, they decided to do IVF with genetic testing. Through two egg retrievals, Brittany got a total of twenty embryos. After genetic testing, she learned that nine were impacted by the syndrome. That left her with eleven embryos, but Brittany still grieved the nine that were discarded.

"Discarding those embryos was devastating for me. I felt so much guilt. I felt like I was abandoning nine little Logans," Brittany said.

The guilt of being a carrier for a genetic syndrome can be so overwhelming. As parents, we hope to pass on our best traits, like big blue eyes or a sharp sense of humor. But sometimes it's a life-changing diagnosis that's passed down. Of course, a parent knows in their heart that they did nothing intentionally to cause their child's diagnosis. Even so, it can be impossible to shake the guilt that comes from knowing their genes contributed to their child's condition.

In the era of advanced medical technology, many carriers turn to fertility treatments and genetic testing to ensure the health of their baby. The process of preimplantation genetic testing (PGT) can be the only hope for carriers to have a child with a normal chromosomal makeup. This act of "playing God" is complex, to say the least, and can evoke mixed emotions about the way we conceive. Regardless of the outcome, the journey is fraught with grief. It's never easy to discard embryos, and this process is emotional, expensive, and heartbreaking.

After four rounds of transfers, Brittany finally became pregnant—with twins. At her eighteen-week appointment, her doctor attempted to commend her for pursuing the genetic testing that ultimately led to a healthy twin pregnancy.

"You did a good job eradicating the mutation," the doctor said.

Brittany audibly gasped as her heart nearly leapt out of her chest.

Eradicating. The. Mutation. Those three words rang out repeatedly in Brittany's mind as she began to think about all the children she knew with rare complexities and how meaningful their lives were. She thought about her son, Logan, and how she wished to hold him in her arms and sing him a lullaby.

Reflecting on all the rare children she had known throughout her life, Brittany said, "It's not about what they accomplish, but how their soul is connected during their time here. I cried in the parking lot that day. I felt like I was abandoning a part of me that was genetically mutated. It felt awful, like something out of a sci-fi movie."

Brittany misses Logan every single day of her life. She's become involved behind the scenes within the rare-disease community, and even though she doesn't currently have a living child who's disabled, she finds connection with Logan through her advocacy work.

In reflecting on how the experience of losing Logan has shaped her, Brittany said, "I wouldn't wish this journey on anyone, but through it, I've found a true lifeline. I've found my people."

One and Done

After giving birth to their disabled daughter, Taylor and Ben intentionally battled against what they perceived as societal pressure to have a big family. Over time, they've noticed how other people react when they say their family is complete with one child.

"When we told my mom that we made this decision, I got the sense that she was disappointed because she wasn't going to get the normal experience. At first, she didn't understand how we could make this choice," Ben said.

Taylor added, "I'm not in the norm having just one kid. It feels like other people expect me to have to have the white picket fence and the perfect life."

Why is this? Why do some people feel uncomfortable with another person's decision to have only one child? Could this go back to the general cultural discomfort with grief and hard feelings? It's hard for loved ones to sit with our (perceived) discomfort and not be able to fix us—in this case, by encouraging us to have another kid. When our loved ones view something as a problem (such as our child's disability), we're forced to live with *their* discomfort. And like Ben said, other family members, like grandparents, might long for a different experience for themselves. But at the end of the day, we as parents must decide for ourselves what is best. We cannot make decisions about our family with other people in mind, especially if the people with opinions aren't going to take an active role in supporting us as parents.

Every couple will have a different journey to reaching a decision about family planning, and Taylor and Ben did not make their decision irrationally. Their daughter, Leah, has a rare variation of Rett syndrome and requires constant care. Taylor has become a full-time caretaker and constant advocate for her daughter.

"We found out about her genetic mutation on the same day we were trying to conceive another baby," Taylor said.

Leah started regressing, ultimately losing the ability to walk independently, and over just a two-week span she lost many of her abilities. The couple ultimately determined that having another child would simply take away from the attention they could give to Leah, and it didn't feel fair to add another child to the mix. They also had to acknowledge that they didn't live near supportive family, and they just didn't have enough bandwidth to raise multiple children. It was then that Taylor and Ben made the decision that their family was complete.

The Decision to Terminate

Kelly was overwhelmed with joy when she discovered she was pregnant after her first round of IUI. She gave birth to a gorgeous boy named Alexander. As Alexander grew, Kelly noticed some developmental delays and quickly got him into an early intervention program. At the same time, Kelly and her husband decided to get pregnant again.

After careful consideration, Kelly opted to have an amniocentesis during her second pregnancy. When the results came back, they were devastating. Kelly's unborn baby had a confirmed chromosomal abnormality. The abnormality was so severe, according to her doctor, that the baby's quality of life was in question.

"There will definitely be cognitive impairment. Beyond that, I don't know. I don't know if she will walk or talk or what her life will look like," the doctor explained.

At the same time, it was clear that Alexander was regressing, although no one quite knew why yet. Kelly began to question whether Alexander might actually be impacted by the same chromosomal abnormality that her unborn baby had. It felt as though overnight Kelly's life began to spin out of control.

After many heartbreaking conversations, Kelly and her husband made the decision to terminate her pregnancy.

The procedure itself was devastating. Kelly wanted a baby. To be more specific, she wanted the baby inside her womb. But her gut told her that something major was going on with Alexander, and she just couldn't fathom having two children with severe disabilities. Kelly followed through with the termination, even though it broke her heart. At the same time, she pursued genetic testing for Alexander, hopeful that it would ease her mind and then she could put this all behind her.

One month after the termination, Kelly and her husband got the results of Alexander's genetic testing. In the blink of an eye, Kelly's entire world as she knew it flipped upside down. Alexander had a rare, degenerative neurological disease. On top of that, he was given an expected life span of twelve years. He was already almost two.

When Kelly reflects on the termination, she feels gratitude for the baby who never made it into her arms. "In a sense, she got my son diagnosed faster and saved me the heartache of having two children with a terminal illness," she said.

Support After Termination

Jessica suffered a heartbreaking loss when she discovered that her unborn baby had multiple holes in its heart and a genetic disorder. Jessica's doctor stressed that the baby was very sick and there was a chance it would not even survive birth. The difficult choice was made to terminate the pregnancy when Jessica was almost nineteen weeks pregnant.

"An abortion of a wanted pregnancy is a huge loss, and it's a unique type of loss because there's an idea that you have a choice. But for many people that I talk to [in a similar situation], their baby is going to die anyway. It's not actually a choice if the baby is going to die," Jessica reflected. Complicating matters further is that abortion laws vary greatly from state to state, and some people must travel long distances to terminate a pregnancy or are forced to carry the child to term.

After the termination, Jessica and her husband found community through a support group specifically for people who had terminated a pregnancy due to medical reasons. "After the first meeting, my husband told me that being part of the group was the first time he'd felt like a real human throughout this entire process," Jessica said.

Jessica now facilitates support groups for people who have terminated a pregnancy due to medical reasons. She has made it part of her life mission to support those who went through a devastating experience like hers.

Jessica's advice to parents who have terminated for medical reasons is to find support once you're ready. "Connecting to other people who had terminated for medical reasons was the only thing that helped me," she said. "I really thought that no one else had experienced this. Once I found support, I was floored to realize that there were other people out there."

Amid the Shame and Pain

There isn't much specific data on termination for medical reasons, but a recent study showed that people who get an abortion for medical reasons are more likely to feel confident about their decision if they have a strong support network. This highlights the need for support during and after a termination, which can be difficult because many people feel uncomfortable sharing news of their termination with others out of fear of judgment. Nevertheless, research supports the benefit of confiding in a close friend who can understand the complex emotions involved in terminating for medical reasons.

There's gratitude, but there's also deep grief and isolation. "There are support groups for loss, but there are none for us. I attended a support group, but it was filled with women who had stillbirths. I couldn't share my story. For a long time, I felt like I couldn't say I terminated the pregnancy. I just said I lost the pregnancy."

• • •

Deciding how many children to have is one of the most important choices a couple will ever make. Parents must be thoughtful about their bandwidths—emotionally, financially, and physically. It takes hard work to show up day after day and balance everyone's needs, including your own. Having a disabled child can shift the family balance because that child may need extra parental support. That said, I encourage you to begin to conceptualize that idea differently. Instead of thinking that your disabled child needs you more, can you begin to see that your disabled child just needs you differently from the way a nondisabled child would need you? At the end of the day, all children need their parents.

If you're looking for permission to grieve the ways in which having a disabled child has changed your expectations for your family structure, know that you're entitled to those feelings. If you feel angry that your carrier status, emotional capacity, or other factors made it so that you needed to limit the number of your children, you're allowed to grieve the choices that were made for you. Within your unique story of parenting a disabled child are likely many sprinkles of grief. When you notice grief coming to the surface, give it air. Grief can never negate the love of your child; you're feeling grief for the loss of how you imagined life would be.

I've yet to meet any parent of a disabled child with high support needs whose family structure wasn't affected by that situation. Whether it's the number of children in the family, the road to conception, or the impact on siblings, having a disabled child in the family can influence nearly everything. The impact, just like disability itself, is multifaceted, complex, life-changing, and rich, and you cannot ignore its presence. I hope you take time to face your emotions and responses to the ways in which your family structure has been shaped by having a disabled child, and that you embrace this experience with compassion—both for yourself and for your family.

Reflection Exercise

Exploring the Four Fs for Your Family

Take some time to reflect on your resources related to the following.

Finances
- Do you feel you could comfortably afford more children with your current income?
- Are there things that could be done to increase your income if you needed to?
- Can you afford additional childcare or would one parent stay home to caretake?

Flexibility

- Would having another child impact the flexibility you need to parent your disabled child? Consider the frequency of hospitalizations, travel for clinical trials, and other appointments.

Fairness

- Do you have the emotional bandwidth to care for multiple children?

- Honestly assess whether it would be fair to your current child(ren) to have more. Can you anticipate any issues that may come up and how you would respond?

Family

- Do you have outsides support? Keep in mind that support is not restricted to family. Support could be a childcare provider, religious community, neighbors, friends, or community resources.

- Would you consider moving to be closer to your sources of support?

- If you need to increase your support network, can you brainstorm ways to do that?

CHAPTER 10

A Whole You

There are many reasons I found myself avoiding writing this chapter. I knew it would be difficult to tie up all the experiences of parenting a disabled child in a pretty little bow without falling back on the clichés and toxic positivity we've all grown so weary of hearing. Pursuing meaningful self-care and connecting to your sense of self is hard, which is why it begins to feel like just another example of the ways in which we're failing to do it all. I often hear parents rattle off statements like "I'm terrible at self-care" or "I don't have the time or money for self-care." I have to ask: Are we truly bad at self-care? Or are we just out of touch with what real self-care is? Perhaps we simply are disconnected from our needs and have a hard time identifying how to refuel ourselves in meaningful ways.

As parents, we spend so much of our brainpower on our kids. We feel guilty if we choose rest over . . . well, pretty much anything. In our modern culture, self-care has turned into a cliché of its own, synonymous with massages, manicures, and wine. But true, meaningful self-care is so much more than an hour of pampering. True self-care leaves you feeling refueled and hopeful—the opposite of burned out. True self-care might look like making a dentist appointment for yourself or going for a walk when you'd rather check out by lying on the couch. Contrary to what modern society tells us, self-care can be hard. It may, at times, not be pleasurable, but it's what we really need to do to feel like we can keep going.

As a therapist and a mom to a child with a disability, Natalie Waybrant has spent much of her career exploring the topic of self-care. "For most of us, self-care feels inaccessible unless we're wealthy. Most of us have never really learned how to practice self-care. For parents of disabled children it's especially hard because as soon as we got that diagnosis, we went into overdrive. It's not until you're able to find some level of stability that you even begin to realize that you've totally lost connection with yourself," Dr. Waybrant said.

Self-care is the first thing that goes out the window when we're in crisis. When our child is in the hospital, there's no time or energy for exercise or connection with friends. During those critical days, we're focused on survival. The pace at which most of us are used to functioning is sustainable for short periods of time, but it becomes problematic when we find ourselves stuck in survival mode long after the imminent threat has passed. For many of us, our early days of caretaking are so demanding that it takes a conscious effort to step out of survival mode.

I remember during Asher's second year of life when my family would make the four-hour drive to my parents' house for the weekend. Suddenly I found myself having extra support. My mom would offer to rock Asher to sleep or take him downstairs to play. I began to notice that it was difficult for me to relax. My brain was stuck in a loop of to-dos and anxiety, even though, for that moment in time, there was actually nothing to be done. My body was also stuck in hypervigilance, which is a key feature of post-traumatic stress disorder. Sitting down and relaxing felt strange to me, and I realized that subconsciously I was afraid of being caught off guard. My brain was convinced that if I let my guard down, something terrible would happen and I wouldn't be prepared. I'm not alone in this experience, as many parents of disabled children report that they feel stuck in survival mode and unable to relax. This is often a sign that our nervous system needs attention, and our body needs to know it is safe.

Calming Your Nervous System

In short, the nervous system makes up your body's communication system. Nerves carry signals and impulses throughout your body. If you've ever touched a hot stove and instantly pulled your hand away, it's because your brain sent an instant message to your body that it was in danger, and your body reacted by moving your hand. Your nervous system includes your brain, spinal cord, and a network of nerves. The goal of the nervous system is to allow the brain to communicate with the rest of your body to keep you alive. Your nervous system has kept you safe in times of crisis, allowing you to jump into action anytime a threat appears. But sometimes the nervous system needs soothing in order for it to recognize that it's safe to return to baseline.

Before you're able to be present enough to benefit from self-care, your body must know that it's safe to put its guard down, which is easier said than done. What makes you feel relaxed? When do you feel safe? What activities bring you joy? Take a moment to answer those questions and connect to the times when your body feels most at ease.

It takes a conscious effort to restore a feeling of safety in your body when you've been stuck in survival mode for a long time. If you notice your heart rate increasing or your anxiety amping up, acknowledge the feeling and then practice a coping skill (see the suggestions in the box on page 194, Effective Ways to Calm Your Nervous System). This is very hard to do when a threat feels like it's constantly looming, such as your child is chronically ill or struggles with uncontrollable behaviors. As hard as it is, you must learn to regulate yourself as much as possible in stressful moments, for your own health and well-being as well as for your child. There will be times when your nervous system kicks into survival mode, but you can learn skills to increase your window of tolerance for stress.

Psychiatrist Daniel Siegel developed the concept of the window of tolerance, which identifies the ideal zone in which you can navigate everyday life. Outside the window of tolerance are the zones of hyper-arousal (heightened emotion, such as anxiety, hypervigilance, panic, anger—this is probably where most parents tend to naturally exist) and hypoarousal (depression, numbness, shame, disconnection). When functioning within the window of tolerance, you are comfortably able to navigate life, even if a few curveballs come our way. Your child comes home from school sick? No problem—you're feeling supported and capable and you can handle this situation calmly. Your child just had a seizure at school and the teacher had to call 911? You're suddenly thrown into the hyperarousal state and flooded with anxiety. When

Effective Ways to Calm Your Nervous System

- Use a weighted blanket. Deep pressure provides the brain with proprioceptive input, which can produce a relaxing effect on the nervous system.

- Snuggle with a loved one or a pet. Snuggling can release endorphins as well as the "love hormone" called oxytocin. This lets your body know it is safe to relax.

- Take a warm bath. Warmth (whether in a bath or via a heating pad, steam room, or sauna) increases endorphins and relaxes your body.

- Meditate or practice yoga. Both meditation and yoga can be hard to sink into when you're stuck in survival mode, but give yourself permission to slow down and focus on your breathing for an extended period of time.

- Practice gentle movement. Go for a walk outside in the sunshine. Put on your headphones if you find that it helps to have something to listen to.

Dysregulated Nervous System

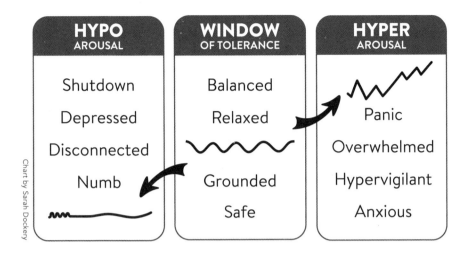

Chart by Sarah Dockery

you're outside your window of tolerance, it's time to call in the coping skills to get you back to sustainable emotional functioning.

I am prone to existing in a state of hyperarousal for far too long (see chapter 7 on health anxiety). When I'm finally able to access self-awareness and notice that I'm highly anxious, I can intentionally reach for some of my skills and prioritize self-care. For me, that looks like spending time outside, snuggling with a pet or loved one, talking it out with a friend, or connecting to people who understand what I'm feeling. These methods are helpful when I need to come back to safety in my body. I have an advantage on the topic of self-care and self-awareness, though, as I spend hours every week as a therapist, helping other people care for themselves. Other parents might struggle to prioritize or even identify how they can care for themselves emotionally.

Meaning Making

In his book *Finding Meaning: The Sixth Stage of Grief*, David Kessler explains that meaning making is the most important stage of grieving. Kessler worked alongside Elisabeth Kübler-Ross in the late 1960s to develop the well-known model of the five stages of grieving: denial, anger, bargaining, depression, and acceptance. But after the death of his son in 2016, Kessler began to understand that acceptance—the former last stage of grieving—wasn't enough. As he grieved the life-changing loss of his son, Kessler began to intuitively search for meaning within the loss to understand how his son's life and death had impacted him.

Finding meaning is not a new concept. Remember back in chapter 2 when we discussed Viktor Frankl and his book *Man's Search for Meaning*? Kessler has expanded on this concept and believes that finding meaning is a necessary skill for surviving life's hardships.

When I first discovered this concept, my instant reaction was skepticism. As a self-proclaimed anti-toxic-positivityist, anything that attempts to force a silver lining is an instant turnoff for me. But upon further examination, it becomes clear that Kessler's addition to the stages of grief is not forcing a silver lining at all. To find meaning in your experience of parenting is simply to ask yourself: How has this changed me? How has raising a disabled child impacted my worldview? How has knowing my child shaped who I am? Finding meaning involves getting to know those little parts of yourself that have bloomed in the aftermath of the hardest thing you've ever done. Instead of fighting against change, you can acknowledge the ways in which parenting has changed you, taking an honest inventory of what is helpful and what is not.

As Asher's mom, I've weathered many storms related to being responsible for his well-being. There have been many times when I've lost sight of who I am in my core. It's easy to drown in a sea of hopelessness and feel like nothing is within my control. I never imagined having a son with a 1-in-20,000 diagnosis. I never imagined having to lock my refrigerator or help bathe my teenage son, who's now taller than me and is beginning to look like a man. There are days I'm so overcome with grief that I feel a million miles away from the person I was twenty years ago, but most days, I know she's still here. I'll hear a song that reminds me of running from stage to stage at Lollapalooza when I was in my early twenties, and I'll remember the hope and optimism I used to have. Or I'll talk to another struggling parent and feel a renewed passion for advocating for parents to be honest about the hard stuff. My sense of self has changed over the years, but the person I was twenty-five, ten, and even five years ago is still a part of me, shaping the very foundation of who I am. Yes, she's changed over the years, but she's been with me all along.

Finding Meaning in Community

Jessica Patay had always been a girl's girl. She cherished her trips with friends and felt most fueled after spending time with the people she loved. Her second son was born with Prader-Willi syndrome, and within two months, she and her husband Chris found solace in a support group for parents of disabled children.

"Community saved me," Jessica said.

Jessica looks back on her early days of parenting her son and feels strongly that she had a calling. "One day I asked myself, what am I going to do with this? What good can I create out of this really hard situation? I know the stress of caregiving. I understand what it's like to not be able to go to the party or on vacation with another family. I started to realize I could make an impact out of my story," Jessica said.

Jessica went on to found We Are Brave Together, a nonprofit that aims to provide community for mothers of disabled children. Jessica and her team have helped launch support groups all over the United States and in New Zealand and Australia. We Are Brave Together offers retreats, connection groups, and many more options for mothers to build community.

"When women come together, they can really support each other. When we leave the cattiness, competition, and comparison behind, the intersection of our lives is a gift," Jessica said.

Jessica channeled her passion for community and friendship into something big by creating We Are Brave Together. She saw a need for a sacred space, led by women for women, where mothers could be vulnerable about their struggles and be supported by people who get it. Perhaps you're reading this and thinking, "I wouldn't even know where to begin with starting a nonprofit." Maybe you're an introvert and that example feels torturous to you. The point isn't that we all need to start nonprofits. The point is that we must create meaning in whatever ways (big or small!) fit with who we are. Jessica Patay always had a passion for community, and she was a natural connector and facilitator. She used her interests and strengths to find meaning in her child's diagnosis in a way that met her grief with compassion, helping not only herself, but many others.

Shifting Priorities

We can find meaning in much smaller ways too. Daniel, dad to a daughter with Sanfilippo syndrome, doesn't plan on ever starting a nonprofit, nor has he made any obvious life changes since becoming the parent to a disabled child. If you didn't know him well, you might not even notice the ways in which he's found meaning through his parenting experience.

Daniel describes his new perspective eloquently, however. "I have learned to cherish every single day with my daughter. Even on the hard days, I try to maintain a sense of levity because I know that someday she won't be here anymore," Daniel said. "There are many days when I feel incredibly sad. None of this is fair and I often get angry about being in this position. But having a daughter with a terminal diagnosis has shown me that life is short and precious. If we want ice cream, we're getting ice cream. There's very little drama in my life and my priorities have definitely shifted."

Finding meaning in your life can be as simple as connecting to your values and worldview. For many of us, having a disabled child shines a giant spotlight on what's most important: health, accessibility, connectedness, community. Finding meaning looks like asking yourself, what are my values and how does my life reflect what's important to me?

Helping Others

Kathryn Knight was faced with a very difficult decision: choosing between leaving her disabled daughter at the hospital for longer than was medically necessary or leaving a job she loved to become her daughter's primary caregiver. Kathryn's daughter was born at twenty-seven weeks and had multiple diagnoses that required a tracheostomy, ventilator, and G-tube. A home health nurse would be necessary to help assist with the tasks of caring for Kathryn's daughter, and Kathryn knew that finding the right nurse would be a difficult task. Kathryn and her husband used social media to spread the word about their nursing needs. Their posts ended up going viral, and the local news aired a segment headlined "Amid an at-home nurse shortage, parents of special needs kids struggle to find help." After the news story ran, nine nurses reached out to the family.

"Our family finally had the nursing coverage we needed, but we also realized that not every family has the incredible luck of securing a news story to help them find nurses," Kathryn said.

Their experience inspired Kathryn's family to found Hello Nurze, a nonprofit resource that allows parents to connect with home health nurses in their community. Parents can create a profile on the organization's website, clearly stating their child's needs and the days and skills that are required. Nurses can then directly message the family and see if they're a good fit. If a nurse and a family connect via Hello Nurze and decide to work together, they can formalize their relationship through a third-party nursing agency of their own choosing. This process keeps the resource free and accessible for all parents.

"We never want any other families to feel the same helplessness we did, and yet we knew there had to be a better way for families to expand their nursing search. This resource didn't exist, so we knew we needed to create it," Kathryn said.

She added, "In the not-too-distant future we expect our daughter will no longer qualify for in-home nursing support because her prognosis is great. However, experiencing the last three years of our journey has truly reinforced how important Hello Nurze is as a resource for medically complex and disability families."

Parenting and Faith

Charlie had a religious upbringing and his faith was an important part of his identity. Through the birth of his disabled son, he has learned to live his life in a less judgmental and more open-minded way.

"There's a huge misconception that just because someone isn't as capable of having a deep conversation over coffee with a friend, their friendships don't mean as much as others' do. Or just because your kid doesn't do hard math in school, their schoolwork is less important than that of other kids," Charlie said.

Having a disabled child has challenged Charlie's view on theology, religion, and ultimately tested his faith in God. "I come from a religious background that tends to be more theological and academic in its principles. While there is a lot of good there, it can be stuffy and elitist at times. When my son got to the age where kids typically start to talk more about their faith, which ultimately leads to them taking communion with the rest of the church, it really didn't occur to me that he would be able to take part in that. Our pastor did a great job of inviting him to be part of that process. He talked to my son like he was any other kid and included us in the process so we could be part of that experience with him," Charlie said.

He went on to explain that he had thought that his son wouldn't be able to participate in the ritual because he might not be able to understand why the church partakes in communion—the theology would be over his head. Thankfully, the pastor at the church explained that faith can be experienced in different ways.

"It's deeply personal. Just because my son experiences faith differently than me and doesn't understand it the same way I might, he still has his own story, journey, and experiences from this that are important to him. This really showed me how biased I was to the way I experience things, and how I don't give others the benefit of the doubt in their own experiences. Not just with disabilities, but with anyone who is different than me—not only can I give them the benefit of the doubt, but I can also learn from how they process and see things differently than me. I can appreciate their journey and know that what is unique about them can be wonderful and life-giving even if I can't relate to it at all," Charlie said.

This is a beautiful example of the intricate and personal ways in which we can find meaning through our child's disability. Charlie's view of faith was widened by his son's existence, which ultimately made him more compassionate and less judgmental. As humans, we learn from other humans. We are softened, challenged, and changed through our parenting experience. Finding meaning through our child's diagnosis can manifest in many different ways; it can be big or small, obvious or subtle, but it's always there.

Finding Purpose

As an architect, Greg Nakata has always been attuned to accessibility in his designs, but it wasn't until he became the father of a disabled child that he realized the unnecessarily astronomical cost of accessibility.

Greg recalls a pivotal moment during a therapy session with his daughter when the therapist presented a switch adapted toy. If you're not familiar with what this means, imagine a stuffed bear where you squeeze the paw and the bear plays music. Squeezing the paw can be difficult for people with certain disabilities, so a bigger button can be added to make the toy more accessible. As it turns out, this adaptation is surprisingly easy to facilitate. The wires just need to be rearranged and connected to a larger switch.

When the therapist showed the toy to Greg's daughter, she began to play with it. Greg, like any parent, was thrilled to see his daughter engaged in play. He immediately set out to get his daughter some adaptive toys to play with at home.

"I got online and saw that the same switch adapted toy the therapist had was $100. And a similar kind of toy was $70. I knew that didn't seem right," he said. Why were these switch adapted toys so expensive?

After receiving one of the toys, Greg quickly took it apart. He found that this toy, which was less than $10 to begin with, was marked up ten times because it included a 40-cent piece that made it more accessible to people with disabilities. This was the moment Greg's passion, AdaptedDesign, was born.

Since tinkering with his first accessible toy, Greg has started an Instagram account, written a book, and created tutorials on how to adapt toys for kids with disabilities. He's even begun adapting items like scissors and knitting tools for disabled adults.

Greg recently connected with a family who had a massive record collection and wanted their disabled son to be able to play records. After some consideration, Greg was able to adapt a record player so that it worked with the touch of a switch and a button. "I love these non-toy things because maybe this child will become a DJ someday. The child is building skills. Maybe record players will be part of his passion someday. It's so cool to me because we are looking beyond toys for kids," Greg said.

Greg's work has grown well beyond toys. He's become an ally to disabled people of all ages and abilities. "Disabled kids will become adults, and they deserve to live in a world where they have autonomy to decide what they want to do. If a record player is that thing, I'm happy to help. I could never put the kind of price tag on toys as other people do. It's about knowing that I'm helping them—not the money," he said.

Greg also reflected on how creating AdaptedDesign has brought him a sense of hope while he navigates his grief about his daughter's continued health struggles. "My daughter was born right before the world shut down for the pandemic, and with her respiratory conditions it was difficult to get out during COVID. We are isolated and don't have a village. I created a community just by posting pictures of switch adaptations. I've made connections all over the country. I still wish we had people close by, but having this community has been amazing. It's given me a purpose."

Creating AdaptedDesign has not erased Greg's grief related to his daughter's health. The pain of watching his child regress and struggle is something that no hobby could alleviate—but the company has brought him joy and a sense that he's doing good in the world.

Finding meaning and acceptance in our experiences is what helps us keep going, even on the hardest of days. It's not a silver lining, but rather a sense of purpose.

When It Feels Impossible

What if you just cannot find meaning in your child's diagnosis? Maybe it feels too overwhelming or sad. I hear from many parents who largely see the world as a darker, more negative place since receiving their child's diagnosis, especially for those with terminal or high-support-need diagnoses. It's easy to see the unfairness in life if you know your child is unlikely to live to adulthood. You may feel alone as you carry the weight of responsibility on your shoulders, and I don't blame you. It's easy to feel like no one fully understands what you're going through. You may be tempted to start seeing the world as all bad and leaning into the isolation you're feeling. Very quickly, you can begin to create your identity around being a victim, believing that only bad things happen to you. The stories we tell ourselves matter. It may be true that you lack support or that your child's diagnosis is devastating, but it's not hopeless. You can begin to find meaning when you're able to tell yourself a new story, a story that honors the nuance and complexities of parenting a child with a disability.

If you find yourself stuck in a hopeless mindset, it's important to consider whether you've lost touch with meaning in life. Where do you find the good? What brings you joy? Of course it's not fair that your child may at times suffer and that you are responsible for caretaking, *and* you cannot lose hope. Both things can be true at the same time. If you're in the trenches and unable to see any good right now, just keep looking. The good is there, and your life (and your child's!) has plenty of meaning. If you can't find meaning, work toward finding acceptance. Acceptance is the first step to finding meaning. This is your (and your child's) life, and you're allowed to feel a wide range of emotions. Your pain and joy coexist.

Through the process of writing this book, I've realized that self-care is closely connected to finding meaning in your child's diagnosis. Meaning fuels your purpose and joy, which in turn gives you a blueprint for self-care. In my case, I'm proud to say I won the graduating class of 2001's writing award at Madison High School (a public school with a class of thirty-nine students, might I add!). Writing has always been a passion of mine. And after I became a therapist and mother to a disabled son, I knew I could be a conduit for other parents to begin to connect to themselves in light of their experiences. Finding my voice started years ago with an awkward post on Instagram in which I shared my vulnerabilities as a parent with my three followers (my husband and my two closest friends). From there, people (strangers, not just people I knew in real life!) joined along and started commenting on my posts and I began to realize I wasn't alone. I wasn't a bad mom for struggling. And a whole lot of parents felt exactly like me; we were all just afraid to say it because we worried that people might think we didn't love our child. I have found meaning in my parenting experience by speaking my truth with self-compassion and inviting other parents to do the same. I used a skill that I've been praised for my entire life (writing) as the medium to make meaning.

You and I both know that you didn't win the Madison High School class of 2001 writing award (because I did), but you have your own passions, worldviews, and values. You have lived your own unique life, shaped by experiences from your childhood, culture, religion, and all the other factors of your story—the good, the bad, the ugly, and everything in between. Parenting a disabled child very well may be your most life-changing experience, but there are many, many other factors that make you who you are. Finding meaning in parenting a disabled child can help you build a bridge from the person you were before your child was born to the person you are now and who you will become. This work can lead you to a choice, reinforce a worldview, make a worldview crumble, or light a fire inside you to create something that makes the world a better place.

The question is, who are you? Who is the whole you, in light of, not in spite of, your role as the parent to a disabled child? Your parenting experience has, no doubt, changed you. But your core self, values, passions, fears, joys—it's all there, and it's important that you give yourself permission to be the whole you as you consider your sense of self and where you find meaning in your life.

I'll never dismiss the hard parts of parenting a disabled child. But with the lowest lows come some of the highest highs. When you've spent endless hours in physical therapy with your child, watching them muster up all their strength to tackle a milestone is earth-shattering in the best way. Seeing your baby smile, make eye contact, come out of a surgery or seizure—these are the moments where you find real meaning in life. On a larger scale, applying your awareness of disability to your worldview can look like realizing that disability is a normal part of diversity and seeing beauty in all people. This is both simple and revolutionary all at the same time.

Being the parent of a disabled child has fundamentally changed the way I view the world. I now understand that all emotions (not just the pleasurable ones) are meant to be a part of life. I now know that the goal is not pleasure. The goal is not perfection. What is the goal? you ask. To be present through all of it. There is so much beauty and value scattered throughout the experience of parenting a disabled child. We get to be a companion to our child through all of life's ups and downs. Parenting is the hardest job. But parenting a disabled child with compassion, advocacy, vulnerability, and balance—that's often the *hardest* hardest job.

We are the keepers of our child's life, often responsible for decision-making and future planning, and not just for eighteen years. It could last one year, or it could last sixty. And if I'm being honest, either option terrifies me. But I can do it, and so can you.

Scattered amid the joy and grief, somewhere under all the care-taking and responsibility, is you. You're not the same person you were before parenting threw your world upside down. You've changed, but you're in there. You're allowed to be more than just a parent. You're allowed to have complex emotions about your parenting experience and not feel like you have to add the caveat "but I love my child so much," because love and pain can coexist.

I've often heard people say something like "take care of yourself; you owe it to your child." But that rhetoric is part of what makes us feel guilty about having complex emotions about parenting. Our child cannot be the sole motivation for our well-being. You deserve to be fully whole, a person who feels all the emotions without self-judgment, a person who advocates for their child and for themselves. You deserve care, love, and self-compassion.

Take care of yourself; you owe it to . . . you.

Reflection Exercise

As you've read this book, you've acquired skills for acknowledging and coping with your emotions, and you've delved into the stories of parents in the trenches of parenting a disabled child. My hope is that these shared experiences make you feel part of a community and less alone in your journey, even if your child's disability differs from those discussed in this book.

Psychologist James Pennebaker's four-day writing protocol, backed by more than 200 peer-reviewed studies, is a powerful tool for improving long-term mental health. This structured exercise asks you to spend fifteen to thirty minutes every day for four consecutive days writing about a challenging issue, and it can be a comforting and effective way to navigate the most difficult aspects of parenting.

By exploring the same challenge for four consecutive days, we begin to find language to discuss a big, scary topic. We untangle the knot and make sense of something that once felt unapproachable. This process gives us the language to confront and process our emotions, leading to changes that can bring more fulfillment and joy into our lives.

In our final reflection exercise, I invite you to commit to Dr. Pennebaker's writing protocol to explore the most challenging parts of your parenting journey. Set a timer for fifteen to thirty minutes and begin to write about your emotions related to parenting a disabled child. Don't worry about your grammar or spelling.

Here are a few prompts you might want to consider:

1. Am I connected to my sense of self?

2. What has been the most challenging part of parenting a disabled child?

3. How has my marriage been impacted by parenting a disabled child?

4. What am I grieving as the parent of a disabled child?

5. How has parenting a disabled child changed me?

6. What do I want to improve in my life?

7. What are my values as the parent of a disabled child, and how can I live my life by them?

Do this exercise four days in a row. Once you've completed the fourth day, reflect on your writings and identify any themes. Notice any common thoughts or feelings. Use the tools you've learned in this book to help you compassionately explore what you need and how to better care for yourself. Give yourself time and gentleness as you begin your authentic self-care and self-compassion journey.

Recommended Reading

Memoirs/Essays on Parenting a Disabled Child

Becoming Brave Together: Heroic, Extraordinary Caregiving Stories from Mothers Hidden in Plain Sight (2024). The Unknown Authors Club.

Dimmitt, M. (2019). *Special: Antidotes to the Obsessions That Come with a Child's Disability.* Ventura Press.

Fein, J. (2024). *Breath Taking: A Memoir of Family, Dreams, and Broken Genes.* Behrman House.

Kim, L. F. (2020). *Can't Breathe: A Memoir.* Paradox.

Lanier, H. (2020). *Raising a Rare Girl: A Memoir.* Penguin Press.

Swenson, K. (2022). *Forever Boy.* Park Row Books.

Disability Support

Coleman, K. (2024). *Everything No One Tells You About Parenting a Disabled Child: Your Guide to the Essential Systems, Services, and Supports.* Hachette Go.

Heumann, J., and Joiner, K. (2020). *Being Heumann. An Unrepentant Memoir of a Disability Rights Activist.* Beacon Press.

Ladau, E. (2021). *Demystifying Disability: What to Know, What to Say, and How to Be an Ally.* Ten Speed Press.

Nakata, G. (2023). *Let's Adapt for Everyone!* AdaptedDesign.

Nielsen, K. (2012). *A Disability History of the United States.* Beacon Press.

Wong, A. (2020). *Disability Visibility: First-Person Stories from the 21st Century.* Vintage.

Yu, T. (2024). *The Anti-Abelist Manifesto: How to Build a Disability-Inclusive World.* Hachette Go.

Therapy/Self-Help

Fradin, K. (2023). *Advanced Parenting: Advice for Helping Kids Through Diagnoses, Differences, and Mental Health Challenges.* Balance.

Frankl, V. E. (2006). *Man's Search for Meaning* (4th ed.). Beacon Press. (Original work published 1946.)

Goodman, W. (2021). *Toxic Positivity: Keeping It Real in a World Obsessed with Being Happy.* HarperOne.

Nagoski, E., and Nagoski, A. (2020). *Burnout: The Secret to Unlocking the Stress Cycle.* Ballantine Books.

Neff, K. D. (2011). *Self-Compassion: The Proven Power of Being Kind to Yourself.* William Morrow.

Pennebaker, J. W., and Evans, J. F. (1997). *Opening Up by Writing It Down: How Expressive Writing Improves Health and Eases Emotional Pain.* Guilford Press.

Siegel, D. J. (2012). *The Developing Mind: How Relationships and the Brain Interact to Shape Who We Are* (2nd ed.). Guilford Press.

Grief

Boss, P. (1999). *Learning to Live with Ambiguous Grief.* Harvard University Press.

Kessler, D. (2019). *Finding Meaning: The Sixth Stage of Grief.* Scribner.

Endnotes

Chapter 1

A 2010 *study discovered that parents of babies who spent time in the NICU* . . . D. S. Lefkowitz, C. Baxt, and J. R. Evans, "Prevalence and Correlates of Posttraumatic Stress and Postpartum Depression in Parents of Infants in the Neonatal Intensive Care Unit (NICU)." *Journal of Clinical Psychology in Medical Settings* 17, no. 3 (2010): 230–237, https://doi.org/10.1007/s10880-010-9202-7.

Research suggests that at least 60 percent of . . . C. Bertsch, "The Course of Acute Stress Disorder and Post Traumatic Stress Disorder in Parents with Infants in the Neonatal Intensive Care Unit," *Dissertations and Theses* (Open Access, 2020): 1007, https://digitalcommons.library.tmc.edu/utgsbs_dissertations/1007

Research shows that scent can conjure up memories . . . R. S. Herz and J. W. Schooler. "A Naturalistic Study of Autobiographical Memories Evoked by Olfactory and Visual Cues: Testing the Proustian Hypothesis," *American Journal of Psychology* 115, no. 1 (2002): 21–32.

Chapter 5

The reality is that disabled people are four . . . P. M. Sullivan and J. F. Knutson, "The Association Between Child Maltreatment and Disabilities in a Hospital-based Epidemiological Study." *Child Abuse and Neglect* 22 (1998): 271–288.

Chapter 7

Study after study underscores the significance of a . . . A. O. Horvath and L. Luborsky, "The Role of the Therapeutic Alliance in Psychotherapy," *Journal of Consulting and Clinical Psychology* 61, no. 4 (1993): 561–573, https://doi.org/10.1037/0022-006X.61.4.561.

Chapter 8

There have been conflicting data over the years . . . E. H. Namkung, J. Song, J. S. Greenberg, M. R. Mailick, and F. J. Floyd, "The Relative Risk of Divorce in Parents of Children with Developmental Disabilities: Impacts of Lifelong Parenting." *American Journal on Intellectual and Developmental Disabilities* 120, no, 6 (2015): 514–526, https://doi.org/10.1352/1944-7558-120.6.514.

Chapter 9

One recent study suggests that growing up . . . Y. Rum, S. Genzer, N. Markovitch, J. Jenkins, A. Perry, and A. Knafo-Noam, "Are There Positive Effects of Having a Sibling with Special Needs? Empathy and Prosociality of Twins of Children with Non-typical Development." *Child Development* 93, no. 4 (2022): 1121–1128, https://doi.org/10.1111/cdev.13740.

Another study suggests that males with a disabled sibling . . . M. Caliendo, V. Lanzara, L. Vetri et al., "Emotional-Behavioral Disorders in Healthy Siblings of Children with Neurodevelopmental Disorders," *Medicina* (*Kaunas*) 56, no. 10 (September 23, 2020): 491. doi: 10.3390/medicina56100491. PMID: 32977671; PMCID: PMC7598646./j.1365-2788.1991.tb00403.x. PMID: 1757979.

Acknowledgments

First and foremost, thank you to my husband, Will. Not only for the extra hours parenting, as I spent many Saturdays writing, but for the ways you've shown me love and patience over our twenty (!) years together. The years spent writing this book were some of the hardest of our marriage because it made me face a lot of feelings I'd prefer to forget. Thank you for your love and forgiveness over the years. It's no secret that you're Asher's person, and you're my person, too.

To my boys, Asher, Silas, and Jasper. You three have always been my why. It is the joy of my life watching you grow up and learning who you are. I will always be here, cheering you on, making you laugh, and embarrassing you. I love you.

To my parents and in-laws, I am forever grateful for your unwavering support. You have been with us every step of the way, sharing our fears and our hopes. Mom, your tender heart for Asher and your willingness to care for him have been a lifeline for us. And Dad, thank you for being the key person and walking Asher to the ambulance as he was transported to the NICU.

As I considered who I wanted to thank for helping this book come to life, I realized I have been surrounded by incredible women who have believed in me, guided me, and encouraged me. First, thank you, Eileen Rosete, for reminding me that this is the book I needed to write and for encouraging me all along the way. Joelle Hann, my developmental editor, thank you for your wisdom and for making this all feel possible when it felt like an impossible dream. Cara Sullivan for the hours you spent reading (and editing!) my book proposal. To Rachel Bennet, thank you for believing in my message early on and always being in my corner. Thank you to Ashley Harris Whaley for having some hard conversations and offering an honest and helpful sensitivity reading.

Kara Baskin, thank you for your graciousness in connecting me to my agent, Jenna Land Free. Jenna, you took a risk on a first-time author and believed in my mission. The stars aligned when my proposal came across your desk, and it really felt like fate connected us. To my editor Maisie Tivnan and our wonderful team at Workman, thank you for your patience and gentleness in this process. You took me under your wing and taught me how to write a book.

To the three who have been there through it all, Liz, Jess, and Lauren. You've cried with me, challenged me, and been with me every step of the way. From the moment Asher was born until this very day—you've been by my side. I would never have had the courage to write this book without your endless encouragement.

And to the many badass women who have supported me and my family over the years and been a model of "what to do when your friend is falling apart"—Jodee, Staci, Jackie, Kassandra, Dana, Kelley, Leigh, Krisi—thank you for being there when it mattered most. To Ms. Kylah and Ms. Angela, thank you for the ways you loved my kids like your own and truly helped mother them while my attention was on writing.

Lastly, to every mom, dad, caregiver, sibling, and therapist who allowed me to interview you, as well as my online community, this book would not exist without you. You've shared your stories with me, allowed me to get to know your kids, and given me so much hope.

Index

About the Author

Amanda Griffith-Atkins is a licensed marriage and family therapist and founder of Amanda Atkins Counseling Group in Chicago. She is passionate about helping parents of disabled children find support and community. As a therapist, she has spent her career focusing on grief, perinatal issues, and couples therapy. Amanda lives in Chicago with her husband, three sons, and a slew of animals.